Cross-Training For Dummies®

Ten Ways to Cross-Train

- **Mix different activities together:** Walk and run; stretch and swim; play softball and go on a hike; lift weights and dance; play Ping-Pong, skate, and use a home fitness video.

- **Use fitness toys:** Exercise with stability balls, exercise bands, balance boards, a step, medicine balls, dumbbells, barbells, weighted bars, weighted vests, and fitness tubing.

- **Create your own mini decathlon:** Try every piece of cardio equipment in the gym — the rower, the stationary bike, the studio cycling bike, the recumbent bike, the Versiclimber, the Stepmill, the step machine, the treadmill, the elliptical cross-trainer, and the arm ergometer.

- **Switch intensities:** Alternate shorter, harder workouts with longer, slower workouts.

- **Work in cycles:** Change what you do, how you do it, and when you do it every workout, every week, every month, and every three months.

- **Do an activity that you've never done before:** Try kayaking, snowshoeing, aerobics, soccer, gymnastics, ballroom dancing, roller hockey, rappelling, or cross country skiing.

- **Multitask.** Do two or more different activities per workout; do three or more different activities per week; do four or more different activities per month; do five or more different activities per year.

- **Shuffle your weight routine:** Change the number of sets, number of reps, order of moves, amount of poundage, and waiting time between sets. Go slower, go faster, couple up moves to superset, and intersperse aerobic intervals with your strength moves.

- **Create diversions mid-workout:** Create an obstacle course during a walk (climb stairs, step up benches, swing off poles, climb over rocks). Add wind sprints during runs. Jump on another cardio machine for 5 minutes in the gym. Add a 5-minute interval, alternating 30 seconds very high and moderate intensity speed or level.

- **Make your strength training functional:** Use lighter-than-usual weights and simulate traditional sports movements — chop, swing, throw, catch, push, punch, pull, and kick.

Tips to Remember When Trying a New Activity

- Bring your sense of humor. It's normal to feel lost, confused, unfit, and uncoordinated.

- Get proper equipment: shoes, gloves, pads, and helmet.

- Learn proper technique from a pro or experienced player.

- Start slowly: Avoid trying to set world records, outmatch your opponents, upstage your instructor, or move/play with perfection your first time out.

- Be realistic about your ability. If you're in good shape, don't push yourself when your skill level isn't up to par. If you're out of shape, don't assume that you're skills are poor.

- Don't do too much, or expect too much, too soon. Since a home run is probably out of the question, a foul is better than a strike, a bunt is better than foul, and a base hit is golden.

- Perfect sports techniques before trying to meet your cardio, strength, and other workout quotas playing.

- Break tricky moves down and hone one component of the skill at a time.

- Commit to at least three sessions before you decide to quit. You never know what hidden talent you have or how much fun what you hated at first can be, but you have to give it time.

For Dummies™: Bestselling Book Series for Beginners

Cross-Training For Dummies®

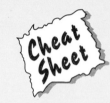

Cheat Sheet

Fitness Lingo You Should Know

cool down: The postexercise phase of a workout, where you gradually decrease the intensity of a vigorous workout to a low intensity.

cross-training: Adding variety to your workouts, either by incorporating two or more types of exercise into one program, or by alternating methods of training to focus on developing different aspects of physical fitness at different periods within a long-term training plan.

endurance training: Doing cardiovascular exercise such as running, cycling, or rowing to improve the ability to exercise for long periods of time.

extension: Opening a joint so that its angle increases, such as when straightening your knee.

flexion: When a joint is bent so that its angle decreases.

high-intensity exercise: Doing cardiovascular or strength exercise at a level that pushes yourself beyond a normal level of exertion.

interval training: A method of alternating very high intensity bouts of activity with rest periods.

ligament: Connective tissue that links bones to each other.

muscle fiber: A single muscle cell.

periodization: Breaking up a long-term workout plan into cycles to alternate different areas of focus.

range of motion: The expanse of movement through which a joint can move.

repetitions: The number of times you perform an exercise within a set.

resistance: The slowing effect (wind, body weight, iron weight, terrain) that must be overcome by force from the muscles.

RPE (Rate of Perceived Excertion): A scale first devised by Swedish Professor Gunnar Borg to rate the level of effort you feel during exercise. The current scale being used is a 10-point scale, with 0 meaning no effort is felt and 10 indicating that the effort is of an extremely high intensity.

set: A group of single repetitions of an exercise.

sprain: When a ligament is torn.

strain: When a muscle or tendon is damaged but not torn.

tendon: The fibrous end of a muscle that connects the muscle to a bone.

Warm-up: The process of slowly raising your heart rate and body temperture at the beginning of an exercise session in preparation to stretch or work up to a higher intensity.

The IDG Books Worldwide logo is a registered trademark under exclusive license to IDG Books Worldwide, Inc., from International Data Group, Inc.
The ...For Dummies logo and For Dummies are trademarks of IDG Books Worldwide, Inc. All other trademarks are the property of their respective owners.

Copyright © 2000 IDG Books Worldwide, Inc. All rights reserved.

Cheat Sheet $2.95 value. Item 5237-6.

For more information about IDG Books, call 1-800-762-2974.

For Dummies™: Bestselling Book Series for Beginners

Praise for Cross-Training For Dummies:

"Finally a book that shows you a no-brainer way to add just enough variety to your exercise program to keep things interesting. If you've had trouble sticking with an exercise routine — like nearly everyone in America — then *Cross-Training For Dummies* is for you."

> — Steven Slon, Editor in Chief, FitLinxx.com

"Martica has a unique ability to give you the science behind the fitness while making it fun to read and easy to understand. In this comprehensive guide to cross-training, she brings together her years of experience as a writer and instructor."

> — Sally Wadyka, Senior Editor, *Women's Sports & Fitness magazine*

"For anyone looking for ideas or motivation, this book is the perfect inspiration to take your fitness routine to the next level."

> — A.J. Hanley, Health Editor, gymamerica.com

"An outstanding how-to book by Martica, one of the fitness industry's most knowledgeable writers. Everybody should use this brilliant guide to train harder, better — and smarter."

> — Nicole Dorsey, M.S., Contributing Fitness Editor for *Oxygen Media*
> and *Parents* magazines

"*Cross-Training For Dummies* is the next best thing to having your own personal trainer. It's filled with motivational tips, techniques, and advice to make sure you're getting the most you can out of every workout."

> — Sarah Mahoney, Editor-in-Chief, *Fitness magazine*

"True fitness is about balance . . . a balanced body, a balanced life. *Cross-Training For Dummies* shows you how to maximize your workouts, so you can reach your fitness goals quickly and effectively, but still have time for living."

> — Kimberly Dawn Neumann, Contributing Writer, *JUMP* magazine

"Finally, a book which provides a safe, easy, effective guide to cross-training! Whether you're a couch potato or avid exerciser, this book is packed with practical, reader-friendly information and guidance which will make working out a breeze. Great for people of all ages, fitness levels, and body types."

> — Hallie Levine, Health and Fitness Writer, *The New York Post*

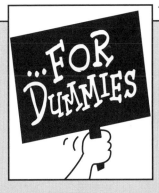

TM

References for the Rest of Us!™

BESTSELLING BOOK SERIES

Do you find that traditional reference books are overloaded with technical details and advice you'll never use? Do you postpone important life decisions because you just don't want to deal with them? Then our *...For Dummies*® business and general reference book series is for you.

...For Dummies business and general reference books are written for those frustrated and hard-working souls who know they aren't dumb, but find that the myriad of personal and business issues and the accompanying horror stories make them feel helpless. *...For Dummies* books use a lighthearted approach, a down-to-earth style, and even cartoons and humorous icons to dispel fears and build confidence. Lighthearted but not lightweight, these books are perfect survival guides to solve your everyday personal and business problems.

> *"More than a publishing phenomenon, 'Dummies' is a sign of the times."*
>
> — The New York Times

> *"...you won't go wrong buying them."*
>
> — Walter Mossberg, Wall Street Journal, on IDG Books' ...For Dummies books

> *"A world of detailed and authoritative information is packed into them..."*
>
> — U.S. News and World Report

Already, millions of satisfied readers agree. They have made *...For Dummies* the #1 introductory level computer book series and a best-selling business book series. They have written asking for more. So, if you're looking for the best and easiest way to learn about business and other general reference topics, look to *...For Dummies* to give you a helping hand.

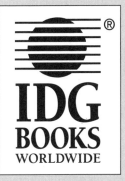

1/99

Cross-Training

FOR

DUMMIES®

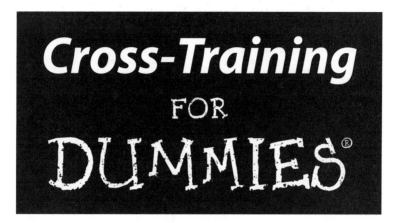

Cross-Training
FOR
DUMMIES®

**by Tony Ryan and
Martica K. Heaner**

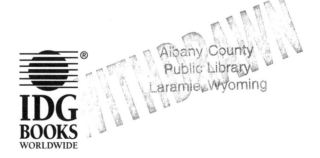

Albany County
Public Library
Laramie, Wyoming

WITHDRAWN

IDG Books Worldwide, Inc.
An International Data Group Company

Foster City, CA ◆ Chicago, IL ◆ Indianapolis, IN ◆ New York, NY

Cross-Training For Dummies®

Published by
IDG Books Worldwide, Inc.
An International Data Group Company
919 E. Hillsdale Blvd.
Suite 400
Foster City, CA 94404
www.idgbooks.com (IDG Books Worldwide Web site)
www.dummies.com (Dummies Press Web site)

Copyright © 2000 IDG Books Worldwide, Inc. All rights reserved. No part of this book, including interior design, cover design, and icons, may be reproduced or transmitted in any form, by any means (electronic, photocopying, recording, or otherwise) without the prior written permission of the publisher.

Library of Congress Control Number: 99-69720

ISBN: 0-7645-5237-6

Printed in the United States of America

10 9 8 7 6 5 4 3 2 1

1O/RQ/QV/QQ/IN

Distributed in the United States by IDG Books Worldwide, Inc.

Distributed by CDG Books Canada Inc. for Canada; by Transworld Publishers Limited in the United Kingdom; by IDG Norge Books for Norway; by IDG Sweden Books for Sweden; by IDG Books Australia Publishing Corporation Pty. Ltd. for Australia and New Zealand; by TransQuest Publishers Pte Ltd. for Singapore, Malaysia, Thailand, Indonesia, and Hong Kong; by Gotop Information Inc. for Taiwan; by ICG Muse, Inc. for Japan; by Intersoft for South Africa; by Eyrolles for France; by International Thomson Publishing for Germany, Austria and Switzerland; by Distribuidora Cuspide for Argentina; by LR International for Brazil; by Galileo Libros for Chile; by Ediciones ZETA S.C.R. Ltda. for Peru; by WS Computer Publishing Corporation, Inc., for the Philippines; by Contemporanea de Ediciones for Venezuela; by Express Computer Distributors for the Caribbean and West Indies; by Micronesia Media Distributor, Inc. for Micronesia; by Chips Computadoras S.A. de C.V. for Mexico; by Editorial Norma de Panama S.A. for Panama; by American Bookshops for Finland.

For general information on IDG Books Worldwide's books in the U.S., please call our Consumer Customer Service department at 800-762-2974. For reseller information, including discounts and premium sales, please call our Reseller Customer Service department at 800-434-3422.

For information on where to purchase IDG Books Worldwide's books outside the U.S., please contact our International Sales department at 317-596-5530 or fax 317-572-4002.

For consumer information on foreign language translations, please contact our Customer Service department at 1-800-434-3422, fax 317-572-4002, or e-mail rights@idgbooks.com.

For information on licensing foreign or domestic rights, please phone +1-650-653-7098.

For sales inquiries and special prices for bulk quantities, please contact our Order Services department at 800-434-3422 or write to the address above.

For information on using IDG Books Worldwide's books in the classroom or for ordering examination copies, please contact our Educational Sales department at 800-434-2086 or fax 317-572-4005.

For press review copies, author interviews, or other publicity information, please contact our Public Relations department at 650-653-7000 or fax 650-653-7500.

For authorization to photocopy items for corporate, personal, or educational use, please contact Copyright Clearance Center, 222 Rosewood Drive, Danvers, MA 01923, or fax 978-750-4470.

LIMIT OF LIABILITY/DISCLAIMER OF WARRANTY: THE PUBLISHER AND AUTHOR HAVE USED THEIR BEST EFFORTS IN PREPARING THIS BOOK. THE PUBLISHER AND AUTHOR MAKE NO REPRESENTATIONS OR WARRANTIES WITH RESPECT TO THE ACCURACY OR COMPLETENESS OF THE CONTENTS OF THIS BOOK AND SPECIFICALLY DISCLAIM ANY IMPLIED WARRANTIES OF MERCHANTABILITY OR FITNESS FOR A PARTICULAR PURPOSE. THERE ARE NO WARRANTIES WHICH EXTEND BEYOND THE DESCRIPTIONS CONTAINED IN THIS PARAGRAPH. NO WARRANTY MAY BE CREATED OR EXTENDED BY SALES REPRESENTATIVES OR WRITTEN SALES MATERIALS. THE ACCURACY AND COMPLETENESS OF THE INFORMATION PROVIDED HEREIN AND THE OPINIONS STATED HEREIN ARE NOT GUARANTEED OR WARRANTED TO PRODUCE ANY PARTICULAR RESULTS, AND THE ADVICE AND STRATEGIES CONTAINED HEREIN MAY NOT BE SUITABLE FOR EVERY INDIVIDUAL. NEITHER THE PUBLISHER NOR AUTHOR SHALL BE LIABLE FOR ANY LOSS OF PROFIT OR ANY OTHER COMMERCIAL DAMAGES, INCLUDING BUT NOT LIMITED TO SPECIAL, INCIDENTAL, CONSEQUENTIAL, OR OTHER DAMAGES.

Trademarks: For Dummies, Dummies Man, A Reference for the Rest of Us!, The Dummies Way, Dummies Daily, and related trade dress are registered trademarks or trademarks of IDG Books Worldwide, Inc. in the United States and other countries, and may not be used without written permission. All other trademarks are the property of their respective owners. IDG Books Worldwide is not associated with any product or vendor mentioned in this book.

is a registered trademark under exclusive license to IDG Books Worldwide, Inc. from International Data Group, Inc.

About the Authors

Martica Heaner: Martica is an award-winning fitness instructor and health writer. She lives in New York City and is the fitness director of *Fitness* Magazine. She teaches classes at New York Sports Clubs, Equinox, and the Peninsula Spa and makes regular appearances as a TV fitness presenter on NBC's *Weekend Today* and other shows.

You might say that cross-training is Martica's middle name. After a childhood spent playing tennis and competitive softball and volleyball in Texas and Arizona, Martica became an aerobics instructor and runner during high school and college. She went to London, England in 1987 to "do Europe" after graduating from college. Instead of traveling, she proceeded to become an integral figure in the development of the British fitness industry. She presented workshops and master classes on choreography and taught techniques to instructors throughout the United Kingdom and Europe. She produced and featured in five fitness videos released in the United Kingdom, including the best-selling *Thighs, Tums, & Bums; SkiFit; Martica's Perfect Curves Workout;* and *Martica's Sexy Body Workout*. She starred in the daily fitness show, *BodyHeat,* which aired in the United Kingdom for 1½ years on L!VE TV. She also wrote over 400 feature articles on fitness, nutrition, and health for newspapers and magazines, including *The Sunday Times* and *The Times* in London, *Fitness, GQ, Men's Health, Shape, Cosmopolitan, Zest, New Woman, Top Sante, Health & Fitness,* and *Fit Body*. She is the author of six other fitness and health books, which were published in the United Kingdom and ten other countries: *Eat More Weigh Less* (1998), *The 7 Minute Sex Secret* (1995), *The Squeeze* (1996), *CURVES—The Body Transformation Strategy* (1995), *Secrets of an Aerobics Instructor* (1994), and *How To Be a Personal Trainer* (1991). She even did a two-year stint as an NFL cheerleader, doing funky dances with pom-poms to stadiums of 15,000 as a member of the Crown Jewels dancers for the European World Football League team, the London Monarchs.

Martica was awarded *National Fitness Leader of the Year* in 1992 based on votes by fitness industry leaders and members of Fitness Professionals, an organization of 20,000 instructors in the United Kingdom and Europe. She was awarded *British Aerobics Champion* (Silver Medal, Mixed Pairs) in 1989 and was nominated for the Special Achievement in the Fitness Industry award in 1993 by the Exercise Association of Great Britain.

She has a Bachelor of Arts in English Literature and Exercise & Sports Studies from Smith College in Massachusetts, and if she ever finishes her master's dissertation on cleft sentences, could have a Master of Arts in Modern English Language from University College, University of London. She has been a fitness instructor and personal trainer for 18 years and is Gold Certified by the American Council on Exercise (ACE) and the Aerobics & Fitness Association of America (AFAA).

Tony Ryan: Tony is a personal trainer in New York City. He is certified by the American Council on Exercise (ACE), and he has a Bachelor of Science degree in Exercise Science from Appalachian State University in North Carolina and an Associate's Degree in Physical Education from Haskell Indian College in Kansas.

He began his love for cross-training in elementary school. "Back then it was called recess. I loved it! Running, jumping, riding, stopping, swinging, and starting again!" Tony realized the potential of cross-training through his high school football coach. Not having the money for fitness equipment, the coach improvised: He would load the football team in a truck and drop them off at a lake five miles away, leaving them with a couple of bikes, a football, a basket-ball, and the order to "dribble, pass, catch, run, walk, or ride back to the fieldhouse within an hour." He had the team push cars around the parking lot: first in neutral, then in first gear, and then in second. And he would have the players jump on each other's backs to do squats and toe raises. During the winter, the team would go to his house and chop wood. Tony continued to play football at Haskell Indian College in Lawrence, KS, where he was also an assistant coach. He went on to play football for Appalachian State University in Boone, NC.

Dedication

From Martica:

To my wonderful, loving grandmother, Beatrice Loock Heaner, who has always given me support and the encouragement to explore the passions in all areas of my life.

From Tony:

To my brother David Bishop. Thank you for waking me up to go to practice. Without you there I wouldn't have. You inspire me.

Authors' Acknowledgments

From Martica:

To Sally Wadyka, Geoffrey Strage, Tamara Chant, and Steven Saltzman: true friends. Throughout this book and beyond, you have always been there to listen or to help out when I've needed you.

To Colleen Esterline, my project editor at IDG with "saint" written into her genetic code. Thank you for your patience, professionalism, and understanding.

To Stacy Collins, acquisitions editor at IDG. We're lucky. You have been more wonderful than words can say. Your diplomacy, humor, and rock-hard glutes are a combination that will take you far.

To my mentors: Sarah Mahoney, my editor-in-chief, and Carla Rohlfing Levy, my executive editor, at *Fitness* Magazine. Thank you for believing in me, supporting me, and giving me such a wonderful reason to cross the Atlantic.

To Mark Reiter at IMG and Tony Ryan. Thank you for enlisting me on the team.

To Richard Cotton, Ph.D. at the American Council on Exercise. Thank you for all your time and helpful advice.

To Wendy Liles, my executive producer on *BodyHeat,* for knowing, just from a phone call, that we were meant to be both professional and personal buddies.

To Darley Anderson, Rowena Webb at Hodder & Stoughton, Brian De'ath at BDP Media, and Ellen Stein. Thank you for all your support over the years.

To Patricia Taylor, M.A., my English teacher at St. Agnes Academy in Houston, TX who gave me the confidence to write. To my exercise physiology professors, James Pivarnik, Ph.D., now at Michigan State University and James Johnson, Ph.D. at Smith College, thank you for providing the inspiration that caused me to make exercise my life. And to Valerie Adams, Ph.D., and Bas Aarts, Ph.D., my linguistics professors at the University of London. Thank you for giving me the opportunity to ponder the meaning of existential *there,* try to make sense of Chomsky's transformational grammar, and realize just how fascinating possessive noun phrases really are.

To my father for understanding everything, and my mother and little big brother, Anthony, for always being there. Finally, is it really silly to thank my kitties, Artichoke and Frederick, who, for all nine years of their lives have shared my lap during every word of every book and every line of every article? Meow.

From Tony:

I am fortunate to have this opportunity to thank all the people that have navigated this book's path with me. This stuff ain't easy, but it didn't kill me so I guess that means I'm much stronger now.

Thank you Jay Kenney for coming back after your first training session. I know it was tough, but it's been two great years since, and I have truly enjoyed every minute of them. Your insights, advice, and friendship have not only made this book possible but made me a better person. There is a lot of you in this book, and I think you'll get a kick out of it.

Mark Reiter, nuthin' but the best for you, my friend. You made it possible for me to share some of the exercise tips and techniques that will help people reach for more in their exercise and in themselves. I don't believe there is a greater gift than that.

When all is said and done, I owe all to the people who have made it really happen. The work that Martica Heaner has put into this book is much appreciated. She definitely deserves a vacation after this one.

Thank you Stacy Collins, for listening to me rant and rave with the patience of a saint. All of you guys at IDG get a big high five and a hug.

To all the coaches, teammates, trainers, and clients that I have had the pleasure of learning from. Thank you from the bottom of my heart. Without all of your instruction, questions, and encouragement, I would not be who I am today. I hope that you get a little something back from the pages in this book.

Last but not least, to my dear friend Doug Joachim. Thanks for putting up with all of this and still being there. Your support means more to me than I could ever say.

ABOUT IDG BOOKS WORLDWIDE

Welcome to the world of IDG Books Worldwide.

IDG Books Worldwide, Inc., is a subsidiary of International Data Group, the world's largest publisher of computer-related information and the leading global provider of information services on information technology. IDG was founded more than 30 years ago by Patrick J. McGovern and now employs more than 9,000 people worldwide. IDG publishes more than 290 computer publications in over 75 countries. More than 90 million people read one or more IDG publications each month.

Launched in 1990, IDG Books Worldwide is today the #1 publisher of best-selling computer books in the United States. We are proud to have received eight awards from the Computer Press Association in recognition of editorial excellence and three from Computer Currents' First Annual Readers' Choice Awards. Our best-selling ...*For Dummies*® series has more than 50 million copies in print with translations in 31 languages. IDG Books Worldwide, through a joint venture with IDG's Hi-Tech Beijing, became the first U.S. publisher to publish a computer book in the People's Republic of China. In record time, IDG Books Worldwide has become the first choice for millions of readers around the world who want to learn how to better manage their businesses.

Our mission is simple: Every one of our books is designed to bring extra value and skill-building instructions to the reader. Our books are written by experts who understand and care about our readers. The knowledge base of our editorial staff comes from years of experience in publishing, education, and journalism — experience we use to produce books to carry us into the new millennium. In short, we care about books, so we attract the best people. We devote special attention to details such as audience, interior design, use of icons, and illustrations. And because we use an efficient process of authoring, editing, and desktop publishing our books electronically, we can spend more time ensuring superior content and less time on the technicalities of making books.

You can count on our commitment to deliver high-quality books at competitive prices on topics you want to read about. At IDG Books Worldwide, we continue in the IDG tradition of delivering quality for more than 30 years. You'll find no better book on a subject than one from IDG Books Worldwide.

John Kilcullen
Chairman and CEO
IDG Books Worldwide, Inc.

Eighth Annual Computer Press Awards ≥1992

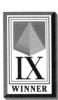

Ninth Annual Computer Press Awards ≥1993

Tenth Annual Computer Press Awards ≥1994

Eleventh Annual Computer Press Awards ≥1995

IDG is the world's leading IT media, research and exposition company. Founded in 1964, IDG had 1997 revenues of $2.05 billion and has more than 9,000 employees worldwide. IDG offers the widest range of media options that reach IT buyers in 75 countries representing 95% of worldwide IT spending. IDG's diverse product and services portfolio spans six key areas including print publishing, online publishing, expositions and conferences, market research, education and training, and global marketing services. More than 90 million people read one or more of IDG's 290 magazines and newspapers, including IDG's leading global brands — Computerworld, PC World, Network World, Macworld and the Channel World family of publications. IDG Books Worldwide is one of the fastest-growing computer book publishers in the world, with more than 700 titles in 36 languages. The "...For Dummies®" series alone has more than 50 million copies in print. IDG offers online users the largest network of technology-specific Web sites around the world through IDG.net (http://www.idg.net), which comprises more than 225 targeted Web sites in 55 countries worldwide. International Data Corporation (IDC) is the world's largest provider of information technology data, analysis and consulting, with research centers in over 41 countries and more than 400 research analysts worldwide. IDG World Expo is a leading producer of more than 168 globally branded conferences and expositions in 35 countries including E3 (Electronic Entertainment Expo), Macworld Expo, ComNet, Windows World Expo, ICE (Internet Commerce Expo), Agenda, DEMO, and Spotlight. IDG's training subsidiary, ExecuTrain, is the world's largest computer training company, with more than 230 locations worldwide and 785 training courses. IDG Marketing Services helps industry-leading IT companies build international brand recognition by developing global integrated marketing programs via IDG's print, online and exposition products worldwide. Further information about the company can be found at www.idg.com.   1/26/00

Publisher's Acknowledgments

We're proud of this book; please register your comments through our IDG Books Worldwide Online Registration Form located at http://my2cents.dummies.com.

Some of the people who helped bring this book to market include the following:

Acquisitions, Editorial, and Media Development

Project Editor: Colleen Williams Esterline

Senior Acquisitions Editor: Stacy S. Collins

Acquisitions Coordinator: Lisa Roule

Technical Editor: Richard Cotton, American Council on Exercise

Editorial Administrator: Michelle Hacker

Editorial Assistant: Beth Parlon

Production

Project Coordinator: E. Shawn Aylsworth, Kristy Nash

Layout and Graphics: Amy Adrian, Joe Bucki, Peter Lippincott, Barry Offringa, Tracy K. Oliver, Jill Piscitelli, Brian Torwelle, Erin Zeltner

Proofreaders: Laura Albert, Corey Bowen, Sharon Duffy, Susan Moritz, Marianne Santy

Indexer: Sharon Duffy

Special Help
Heather Prince, acquisitions coordinator; Arthur Belebeau, photographer Amanda Foxworth

---

General and Administrative

IDG Books Worldwide, Inc.: John Kilcullen, CEO

IDG Books Technology Publishing Group: Richard Swadley, Senior Vice President and Publisher; Walter R. Bruce III, Vice President and Publisher; Joseph Wikert, Vice President and Publisher; Mary Bednarek, Vice President and Director, Product Development; Andy Cummings, Publishing Director, General User Group; Mary C. Corder, Editorial Director; Barry Pruett, Publishing Director

IDG Books Consumer Publishing Group: Roland Elgey, Senior Vice President and Publisher; Kathleen A. Welton, Vice President and Publisher; Kevin Thornton, Acquisitions Manager; Kristin A. Cocks, Editorial Director

IDG Books Internet Publishing Group: Brenda McLaughlin, Senior Vice President and Publisher; Sofia Marchant, Online Marketing Manager

IDG Books Production for Branded Press: Debbie Stailey, Director of Production; Cindy L. Phipps, Manager of Project Coordination, Production Proofreading, and Indexing; Tony Augsburger, Manager of Prepress, Reprints, and Systems; Laura Carpenter, Production Control Manager; Shelley Lea, Supervisor of Graphics and Design; Debbie J. Gates, Production Systems Specialist; Robert Springer, Supervisor of Proofreading; Kathie Schutte, Production Supervisor

Packaging and Book Design: Patty Page, Manager, Promotions Marketing

◆

The publisher would like to give special thanks to Patrick J. McGovern, without whom this book would not have been possible.

◆

Contents at a Glance

Cartoons at a Glance

By Rich Tennant

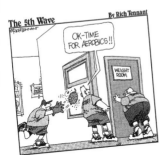

page 9

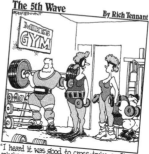

"I heard it was good to cross-train, so I'm mixing my weight training with scuba diving."

page 35

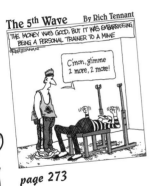

page 273

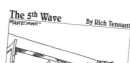
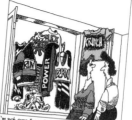

page 89

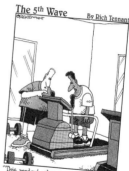

"This readout shows your heart rate, blood pressure, bone density, skin hydration, plaque buildup, liver function, and expected lifetime."

page 301

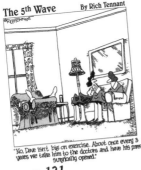

"No, Dave isn't big on exercise. About once every 3 years we take him to the doctors and have his pores surgically opened."

page 121

"I'm not sure I can live up to my workout clothes."

page 235

Fax: 978-546-7747
E-mail: richtennant@the5thwave.com
World Wide Web: www.the5thwave.com

Table of Contents

THE INFORMATION IN THIS REFERENCE IS NOT INTENDED TO SUBSTITUTE FOR EXPERT MEDICAL ADVICE OR TREATMENT; IT IS DESIGNED TO HELP YOU MAKE INFORMED CHOICES. BECAUSE EACH INDIVIDUAL IS UNIQUE, A PHYSICIAN MUST DIAGNOSE CONDITIONS AND SUPERVISE TREATMENTS FOR EACH INDIVIDUAL HEALTH PROBLEM. IF AN INDIVIDUAL IS UNDER A DOCTOR'S CARE AND RECEIVES ADVICE CONTRARY TO INFORMATION PROVIDED IN THIS REFERENCE, THE DOCTOR'S ADVICE SHOULD BE FOLLOWED, AS IT IS BASED ON THE UNIQUE CHARACTERISTICS OF THAT INDIVIDUAL.

Introduction

· ·

*A*nyone can get into a fitness rut. You could be exercising regularly but feeling unmotivated by your current routine. Or you could be enjoying your workouts but not getting the results you really want. You can even be on a health club hiatus and looking for a way to get back into exercise-mode.

Let cross-training come to the rescue. Cross-training is a way of varying your workouts. It can be as simple as trying something new by venturing out of your comfort zone (or familiar activity) to pick up a ball, hop on a bike, or pump weights. Or it can be a way of planning and organizing your exercise sessions to focus on different goals at different times so that you improve specific skills or overall performance in different sports or activities. While we can't promise that cross-training will cure world hunger or help the New York Mets win the World Series, it may be just the thing you've been looking for — a way to inject a little excitement and better results into your exercise plan. If any of the following apply to you, cross-training is the solution you need:

- ✔ You're in good shape, but good is not enough: You want to do something more.
- ✔ You find exercise boring, boring, boring (and that's why you don't do it as much as you should).
- ✔ Your current workouts that used to have you counting the minutes until your next visit to the gym have become a predictable chore and something you'd rather ignore.
- ✔ You do the same activity over and over . . . and have an injury, or a hint of a weakness, that simply won't go away.
- ✔ You want to challenge yourself to greater fitness heights because advanced fitness classes and weekend football in the park just don't do it for you anymore.
- ✔ You want a better butt, stronger arms, or a flatter gut.
- ✔ You know that *how* you do what you do is key and you want to learn how to exercise with better technique.
- ✔ You're not getting the results you want.
- ✔ You want to take your body to the next level: from ho-hum to fit, or from fit to goal-scoring glory.

Enter cross-training . . . the jumpstart you need for your health, heart, and happiness!

Cross-training is a well-rounded way of approaching exercise. In the most basic sense, it's simply varying your workouts. Instead of just running three days a week, you might also bike and swim. Or instead of just using the step machine at the gym, you might also use the rower and the treadmill or do a weights circuit during your session.

In the more technical, sports-specific sense, cross-training is a strategic approach to training. You vary your exercise schedule in order to develop specific skills or aspects of fitness that will enhance your performance in a specific activity or sport. If you were to apply a cross-training plan to your running schedule in order to train for a marathon, you might alternate periods of working on running speed and distances, as well as incorporate a strength training and flexibility program. To cross-train to improve your performance when playing basketball, you might start with a period of developing basic cardio fitness and then focus on exercises to enhance your sprinting speed across the court and your free throw accuracy. Either way you do it, cross-training will keep you interested, motivated, strong, and (if you listen to your body) injury-free.

About This Book

If you have a real thirst for fitness knowledge, grab a sports drink, cuddle up next to your treadmill, and read every word of this book to soak up the fitness wisdom that we've culled from a combined 29 years in the fitness industry. We've trained people of all sizes and shapes at fitness levels ranging from downright slobular to sports superstardom. In those years, we've learned a thing or two about what works (and what doesn't), and we're going to share our knowledge with you. Plus, we include lots of interesting stuff about the way your body operates that you might just find as fascinating as we do.

You can use this book in several ways:

 ✔ If you've been working out, but you don't feel comfortable with the terminology everyone's using or you just don't know where to start, begin reading in Part I. You can try the Fitness Tests in Chapter 5; they will help assess your level of fitness and the areas where you may be weak, but you should see a doctor and/or fitness professional to make sure your body is ready for action.

 ✔ If the gym is a place where everyone knows your name, you may want to skip on over to Part II, where you set your fitness objectives and analyze your current fitness level. After that, you can hop over to the Cross-Training Plans in Part III to find one that matches your motives (to lose weight or train better for a certain sport, for example). Find the exercises you need to follow for your plan in Parts IV and V, and get moving!

✔ If you tend to be an organized/clean desk kind of person (one sure sign: you're a compulsive list-maker), taking cross-training *seriously* might be just the thing you need to get more interactive with your workouts. You'll love the concept of *periodization,* which we explain in Chapter 3; you can plan, schedule, and organize your workouts to your heart's content.

✔ When you've finished your first 12-week plan, evaluate your progress by retaking the Fitness Tests in Chapter 5 and reassessing your goals. Ready to mix it up? Go back to the Cross-Training Plans in Part III, and modify your existing plan to make it more challenging, try a new one, or create one of your own.

✔ You can come back to this book again and again to find new ways to cross-train. Just scan the table of contents or index to find a topic that'll motivate and inspire you with new insights.

Challenging your body to new fitness levels is hard work, so no matter how you begin, please take time to read the guidelines in Chapter 6 concerning your health and safety, as well as the tips on listening to your body in Chapter 13. You should see your doctor before embarking on one of the cross-training programs in this book or any new fitness program. Seek out help from a doctor if you have any questions in regard to skeletal, muscular, cardiovascular, and orthopedic conditions.

Foolish Assumptions

We have to let you in on a little secret: The training tips in this book are not suitable for everyone who picks it up. If you've been working out for a while, are relatively fit, and are looking for something to challenge you, you're going to love what we have in store for you. While we have a lot of options for ultra beginners, you may want to check out *Fitness For Dummies,* 2nd Edition, by Suzanne Schlosberg and Liz Neporent or *Workouts For Dummies,* by Tamilee Webb and Lori Seeger (both from IDG Books Worldwide, Inc.) before stepping up to the cross-training plate.

How This Book Is Organized

Cross-Training For Dummies is divided into seven parts. The first two parts explain in detail how cross-training works and all the things about fitness that you should understand — from how to set goals, how your body gets stronger, and how to keep your workouts as energetic and effective as possible. Part III gives you step-by-step plans that you can follow — starting today (literally), you can plug in the activities you already do into one of these pre-formed, well-balanced training programs. We've done all the thinking for you, so that all you have to do is just do it (thanks, Nike). Parts IV and V are a virtual exercise bible with a breakdown of over 75 exercises that you can do to work each and every body part (even those you didn't know existed). We include drills, skills, and muscle strengtheners. This reference guide — to everything from the most basic to the most challenging exercise you should do — is something you'll want to refer to for years to come (we hope). Finally, in Part VI we give our assorted Part of Tens chapters, offering tidbits that will help you stay inspired, such as motivation tips, fascinating facts about muscles, and a whole-body stretch routine that you can do on a bench, bed, or couch. Remember to check out the Appendixes where you'll find a blank, ready-to-use workout log; a comprehensive list of product manufacturers, fitness associations, and other contacts for all your fitness needs; and a glossary that you can refer to for quick definitions of technical fitness terms.

Part I: Wake Up Your Workouts

Variety is the spice of your exercise life. In this part we explain what happens if you do too much of the same thing and/or stick to the status quo (not good, trust us).

Part II: Let's Get Specific

Your exercise program is as precise as a recipe: What you do with the ingredients you add determines your results. In this part we steer you to the right part of the cookbook for your body and your goals. We show you how to personalize your program by figuring out what areas you need to improve and what to focus on to be successful. And we also show you how to approach your workouts as safely as possible.

We get down to the cool details that explain, for example, why some people should work harder than others, why some ways of exercising don't do what you think they're doing, and how different ways of exercising can maximize your energy levels.

Part III: Cross-Training Plans

Do you want to lose weight without too much foot-pounding or hard work? Or do you want to excel at a sport like running, cycling, or your after-work softball team? We give you a series of plans to choose from that will help you to reach your goals.

Part IV: Fabulous Moves

Whether you're a complete beginner to strength exercises or you've been doing the same basic moves for years, we show you how to refine your exercise technique. First, we take a new look at some old moves — make sure not to skip this because it's old hat; you may have fallen into sloppy habits because you're *too* familiar with a basic abdominal or leg exercise. We pinpoint how to perfect your form, and then we give you lots of new variations of upper and lower body exercises to keep your muscle fibers (and brain) stimulated. This part also steers you to some tough sports moves that will develop your power and coordination.

For every single exercise, we show you the proper alignment and tell you how to focus on the muscles you're working. And we give you important safety tips so that you get stronger, not weaker, from these moves!

Part V: Move That Body!

Here's a breakdown of the range of sports and other activities that you can incorporate into your workouts. We explain key things you should think about, including what results you can expect and how best to prevent injuries. We include everything from fitness classes to team sports. Hopefully this section will also inspire you to try something new as you plug in activities into your cross-training program.

Part VI: The Part of Tens

We don't think you'll tire of cross-training very easily since the ever-changing variables of your workouts will keep you on your toes. But let's face it, we all slack off at some time or another. Here we give you ten ways to stick to your program. We also include ten things you should know about your muscles and ten great bench stretches.

Part VII: Appendixes

Since keeping track of what you do can be a key motivating tool that will keep you committed, we include a workout log to help you monitor your progress. We also include a thorough list of contacts, where you can learn more about cross-training and other forms of getting in shape. You can keep your flexibility training fresh by using some of the bench stretches we give you here in place of the stretches in Chapter 15.

Icons Used in This Book

We know you're busy. So to make sure that you can get what you want from this book *quickly,* we flag key points by sticking little icons next to them. So as you leaf through you'll know to pay special attention if you'd like more practical advice on how to perform your workouts. Check out the icons to see what you're most likely to want to notice.

 Your body is a machine with lots of fascinating parts. When we detail the scientific stuff you might want to know, we alert you with the Technical Stuff icon.

 We use the Warning bomb to alert you to an exercise or way of training that can result in injuries.

 Our Tip target points you in the best direction to get the most from an exercise or training method.

 Thanks to the continuing research efforts of exercise physiologists and other scientific exercise-types, what you may have learned as fact in gym class, or even last week at the gym, might now be fiction. Even traditional ways of training might have new caveats that you should be aware of. The Myth Buster superhero keeps you exercise-savvy.

 Tony's enthusiasm about exercise is infectious, and Martica's insights will help you take a more intelligent approach to exercise. Check out these sections for both trainers' tips, tricks, and techniques.

Special Icons

Look for these special icons in Parts III, IV, and V, which direct you to the various elements of fitness:

 The Cardio Stamina icon points to exercises that will work your heart as well as your whole body.

Looking for moves that strengthen your muscles and the joints that support them? The Muscle Strength icon can show you where to go.

The Power icon usually hangs around its sporting buddies because they go hand in hand. When you see it, you'll know that it wants to add power to your workouts.

If you see the Flexibility icon, be on the lookout for moves that will help keep you limber and loose.

The Skills icon points to activities that emphasize speed, agility, and coordination.

Where to Go from Here

You're ready to roll (or walk, run, or skate). Start at the beginning, or flip to Part III to find a Cross-Training Plan that suits you. Parts IV and V introduce you to the exercises you'll find in the Cross-Training Plans. You can also use the table of contents and index to find specific topics. (See the "About This Book" section earlier for some suggestions on getting you started.)

When you're ready to follow the plans and dive into the exercises, get a doctor's okay first before you start.

> THE INFORMATION IN THIS REFERENCE IS NOT INTENDED TO SUB-STITUTE FOR EXPERT MEDICAL ADVICE OR TREATMENT; IT IS DESIGNED TO HELP YOU MAKE INFORMED CHOICES. BECAUSE EACH INDIVIDUAL IS UNIQUE, A PHYSICIAN MUST DIAGNOSE CONDITIONS AND SUPERVISE TREATMENTS FOR EACH INDIVIDUAL HEALTH PROBLEM. IF AN INDIVIDUAL IS UNDER A DOCTOR'S CARE AND RECEIVES ADVICE CONTRARY TO INFORMATION PROVIDED IN THIS REFERENCE, THE DOCTOR'S ADVICE SHOULD BE FOLLOWED, AS IT IS BASED ON THE UNIQUE CHARACTERISTICS OF THAT INDIVIDUAL.

Part I
Wake Up Your Workouts

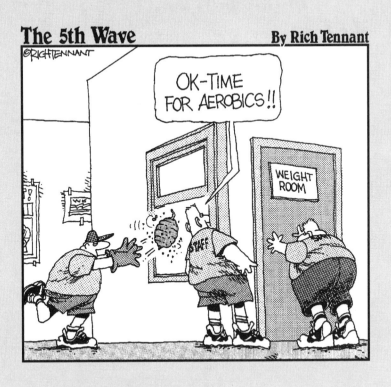

In this part . . .

We look at why you need to add pizzazz to your fitness routine. (And we take a sneak peak into the future to guesstimate what will happen if you don't.) This part introduces the concept of intelligent training — how to plan and balance out your workouts. We'll show why just aiming for a better butt isn't enough to get you one or why *just* running or *just* doing ab crunches isn't the most effective way to improve your strength, stamina, and skills for each activity. Striving for total, all-over fitness will get you the best looking, best performing body ever.

Chapter 1

Your Ever-Changing Body

*1*n times gone by, chopping, grinding, lugging, pulling, plowing, sowing, and hunting and gathering were activities that the human body had no choice but to perform. This total body living gave the arms, legs, back, abs, and other body parts a real-life cross-training workout every day. Things have changed. Now, tapping the remote control, twisting the ignition, or taking a long stretch to answer the phone are about the extent of the activity that we do. And for all the health reasons that we already know, as this century leaves us with too many opportunities to plant ourselves in increasingly sedentary lives, it's vitally important that we use exercise as a replacement for the daily chores that we were once required to do.

We know that as a sometime exercise fanatic at least *a little bit* of your time is spent away from the boob tube and logged off of the Web in pursuit of a work-out. It just might not be as often as would like (or need to). Even if you've made exercise a habit in your everyday schedule (good), your workouts may have become a habit (bad). No one's immune to the temptations of slothdom or the trap of boredom. Everybody needs a push, and we mean *every body*. The human body thrives on being asked to go past its normal comfort zone in terms of how much energy, force, and physical skills it's required to use. That's where we come in, your personal cross-trainers at your service, to offer fitness tips, tricks, and advice. We're here to push you to the next fitness level.

This chapter tells you why what you're doing now may not be enough. Cross-training has multiple benefits, as you'll see in this chapter. The last section of the chapter presents the general steps you'll follow in creating an exercise program that works just for you.

The Pitfalls of Status Quo

Picture a cute little bunny rabbit in the wild. In order to stay alive, he needs to adapt to the changes in the environment. If he doesn't hop around enough, he won't find food. He might become slow, weak, and unable to run from the mean fox trying to eat him. We're like that bunny — all the living, growing organs in our body, from skin to muscles to blood, react to the stressors they are exposed to. So when things get tough, remember that you get more resilient with controlled, challenging doses of stress. To become stronger, longer lasting, or more flexible, the body adapts in its multitude of physiological ways (from releasing tension to growing more muscle or improving nerve signals from brain to body part in order to get stronger).

Any type of exercise you do is a stimulus to get these improvement processes underway. But once you've been doing the same routine, or exercising at the same intensity, for a while, your body grows accustomed to the challenge, meets it, and beats it. Soon, what was adequate stimulus for growth becomes a normal level of physical effort. It's not that the same-old, same-old exercise stops working. It's that, once you're capable of handling it, to continue to do the same workout in the same way simply maintains, but doesn't improve, your level of fitness.

And for some people that's fine. If you're simply exercising as a form of stress relief or to improve your long-term health, you're probably okay just staying active and enjoying what you do. But if you're trying to lose weight, reshape your body, or dramatically improve your physical performance in a specific activity, you need to approach your training with a plan. And that's where this book comes in.

Cross-Training Is Intelligent Training

Cross-training is a way to add variety — and constant new challenges — to your workouts, and it targets your whole body. Here are a few of its best benefits:

- **Less burnout:** Because you'll constantly be incorporating new exercises, sports, and activities into your routine, you'll be less likely to suffer from burnout and quit.

- **Fewer injuries:** Cross-training is a great way to make your body as efficient as possible, while keeping it almost injury-free. By switching activities, you vary the stresses on your body. This often means less injury risk because most fitness injuries are due to overuse (doing the same thing over and over) and the repetitive strain of a given movement.

✔ **Benefits your whole body:** Chapter 2 covers the benefits of cross-training on your whole body. Cross-training can improve your cardio stamina, muscle strength, power, flexibility, and sports skills.

✔ **Better performance in sports:** You also can gain a better all-around fitness because you're not just developing a specific ability in one activity but in a number of them. For example, rowing may develop your upper body while cycling favors the lower body. Weight training can give you all-over muscular strength that running alone simply cannot.

✔ **More calories burned:** You may also burn more calories. Since your body responds to exercise by getting more efficient at producing energy for an activity, you ultimately push yourself less and burn fewer calories once your body has adapted. When you cross-train, because your body is always adapting to new forms of stress, it keeps working hard to keep up.

Cross-Training Is Full of Choices

The way you cross-train can vary immensely. It provides you with options on a daily, weekly, monthly, and yearly schedule. To help you get a little background, here's an outline that can help you wade through by directing you to the areas in the book where you'll find more information about each decision you must make:

1. **Evaluate your level of fitness and your goals.**

   What do you want to get out of cross-training? Are you wanting to try new ways of working out or looking for ways to hit peak performance? Part II presents you with some goal setting tips of the trade. Then read on to evaluate your level of fitness using the at-home fitness tests we provide. (***Remember:*** You should always get your doctor's okay before embarking on a new fitness program.)

2. **Pick a plan to follow from Part III, or create a plan of your own.**

   Part III has three plans that are real no-brainers. Just choose one and get moving. You can also create your own plan by following the suggestions in Chapter 12.

3. **Mix things up with your daily and weekly workouts.**

   Just because you're following one of the plans in Part III doesn't mean you can't add variations on your own. Cross-training is all about mixing things up, as you'll see in Chapter 3.

   You can mix two or three different activities into each workout (see Chapter 3) or incorporate different activities within your regular weekly routine (Monday: run, Tuesday: walk up hills, Wednesday and Friday: take a body sculpting class).

You can get technical by choosing different areas to train for, such as flexibility, muscular strength, and coordination (see Chapter 2 for an introduction to these topics). You can also rotate high and low impact sports, high and low intensity activities, and simple-to-complex movement patterns.

4. **Let your Type A personality take over and plan a month or year in advance!**

   You must be thinking we are crazy, but athletes create long-term plans all the time! Athletes use *periodization,* which is a system of creating a long-term schedule of training cycles that focus on developing different aspects of fitness that will improve performance. You discover this in Chapter 2.

   And you'll know where you're going because you'll be tracking your progress all along the way. Remember the fitness tests in Step 1? Well, every 12 weeks you should re-evaluate yourself. This way, you'll have an idea of what things you can do to push yourself the next time around.

You're an all-star athlete

The concept of cross-training is nothing new. It was made popular with the advent of triathlons — endurance competitions where you run, bike, and swim in one race. But cross-training is important, and if you're not doing it already, we're here to show you how. Here are a few examples of activities, what they do and do not do for you, and what you can incorporate into your routine to get a thorough, balanced workout:

What Activity You Do Now	Fitness Result	What It's Lacking	Activity You Should Cross-Train With
Running	Cardio stamina	Flexibility	Stretching
Yoga	Flexibility	Strength, cardio	Weights, cardio
Sculpting	Strength	Cardio	Sports, aerobics
Football	Sports skills, cardio	Flexibility, strength	Stretching, weights

If you're an athlete training for a certain sport, you may cross-train with a highly planned out schedule. So, in addition to your main sport, you phase in a different activity for a number of weeks and then add another new one to improve all the physical attributes you'll need to excel at your sport. Check out Chapter 11 for the Athletic Plan.

Chapter 2

A Rock-Hard Rear Is Not Enough

● ●

In This Chapter

▶ Benefiting your whole body

▶ Using food as fuel

▶ Presenting the elements of exercise

● ●

Getting fit is not as easy as choosing a few body parts to target and forgetting the rest. Yet some people approach their workouts like this. Some women exercise their butt and thighs to death but neglect their drooping back, arm, and shoulder muscles. Some men pummel away at their bellies and pecs but let their chicken legs go untouched. Some athletes practice running or throwing for hours but neglect stretching and strength work. Some people are committed exercisers, but they eat so much junk food that they starve themselves of precious nutrients that are vital for a healthy, efficient body.

To achieve total fitness for your whole body, you must combine moves and activities that constitute a wide range of movement patterns, exercise intensities, and modes of exercise. Getting the right combination can seem daunting, especially for the beginning exerciser. Fortunately, cross-training helps to click these puzzle pieces into place. Remember that what you eat is an important part of the equation. No matter how well you train, it's the nutrient-packed foods that allow your body to function at its optimum.

This chapter covers how your body uses the food you eat for energy. It then introduces the pieces of the fitness puzzle — cardio stamina, muscle strength, power, flexibility, and sports skills — and jargon you need to know to get yourself into the best shape ever!

Focus on the Whole Body

Although many of our clients and students come to us to improve their health and athletic abilities, a majority of them focus on trying to look better. Looking better isn't a matter of identifying your "problem area" and then focusing on that. Good looks are about body symmetry. You can have the most attractive arms, abs, or face in the world, but if you're hunched or slumped, your good bits aren't as noticeable.

Not only can focusing on just a few areas of fitness or a few muscle groups make you look unproportioned, it can also create muscular and fitness imbalances. Muscles provide stability and support for the skeleton and work synergistically to perform various movements. Their overall alignment is a complex balance of strength and flexibility. If one area of the body is weaker, postural and other imbalances can occur and lead to serious injuries. If you've developed one aspect of fitness, such as your cardiovascular stamina, but neglected another, such as strength or coordination, it can affect your performance.

Tony likes to emphasize that you're only as strong as your weakest link. There's no sense overworking one thing and underworking another. Your strongest area of fitness is likely to be inhibited by the weaker areas, so you're better off training your whole body.

A balanced body also gives you confidence, and confidence is the key ingredient not only to succeeding in a sport — you'll be aggressive in making game-changing plays — but in your personal life as well. Confidence is sexy! Tony had a client, Bob, who wanted to improve his cycling performance. After a period of regular sessions, Bob's body got stronger and his thighs blossomed from spindly pencil legs to voluptuous powerhouses. He started beating his best times in cycling events, and he even got the girl — he met and married a professional cyclist.

Revving Your Body's Engine

You eat a banana. You start to run. What must happen to give you that energy? Your body gets into high gear and starts putting its energy systems to the test. You're a metabolic miracle, and if you've never been interested in mechanics before, listen up: Your body is a fascinating machine.

Energy = Fat + Carbs + Protein

Like a rock band with longevity, your body moves and grooves with the times. Your body reacts differently depending upon how it moves because it requires different levels of energy. It can move slowly, at a moderate pace, or very fast. It can move for just a few seconds or several hours. You can use a few, or many, muscles to produce the movement. The muscles might have to exert very little force in order to move, such as when walking. Or they might have to work extra hard against different levels of resistance (from walking uphill, cycling in wind, or moving a heavy weight). All the different combinations of these variables affect how the body gets the energy to make the movement possible.

Without getting too technical about chemicals, we'll just say the body relies on two main fuel sources: fat and carbohydrates. Protein is a back-up energy source used when the body is in starvation mode. (Despite what muscle-bound bodybuilders used to believe when they chugged down gallons of protein drinks or what some trendy high-protein diet plans like to promote, protein is definitely not the energy source we rely on for exercise.) The unit used to measure energy is a calorie. There are fat calories and carbohydrate calories, and both give your body energy.

✔ *Carbohydrates* and the other quick energy sources in the body are like kindling and paper. They burn quickly, so when you need to increase your metabolism fast (like when you get up off your chair and start walking quickly), it makes sense for the body to consume energy from this fuel source. But limited stores of this type of energy are available in the body, so if the exercise is to continue for some time, it's more efficient for the body to rely on its fat for fuel.

✔ *Fat* is like coal: It burns slowly and lasts a long time. Plus, (and we know this might not be good news to you) you have billions of fat cells in your body. Look on the bright side! This means you have endless stores of fat fuel that your body can use for energy. Because fat is so efficient, the body will naturally shift to a greater emphasis on fat burning for fuel the longer exercise continues in any one session. However, even though you're burning a higher percentage of fat the longer you do an aerobic activity, you're still burning carbs, too. In fact, if your carbs weren't being used, you wouldn't be able to metabolize fat because fat burns in a carbohydrate flame.

If you've ever heard of marathoners "hitting the wall," it's because they have exhausted most of their carbohydrate stores during their run, usually after about 22 miles. While at this stage in the run — some two or three hours (or more) into it — they are in high fat-burning mode, their carbohydrates are still being used — and slowly being depleted. As you get fitter from a training program of regular exercise sessions, one of the many ways that your body improves is that it learns to use a greater percentage of fat during both intense and long duration activities. This allows you to conserve some of your carbs during intense movement, allowing you to last longer.

Great myths of fat burning

Judging by all the informercials, diet pills, and other products offering to zap the fat from your body, fat burning is a coveted thing. When your body churns to draw upon the energy needed to move around, whether it uses more fat or more carbs depends on the intensity of what you do. But when it comes to losing weight, calories are calories and the distinction between which kind of calories are used isn't that important. You're fat burning when you're in couch-potato mode, for goodness sakes. Yet, a lot of misunderstanding prevails.

Here we break down some of the myths people have about burning fat:

- **Myth:** The body completely shuts off one fuel source when it turns on the other.

  The Truth: What has often been misunderstood by both exercisers and exercise instructors alike is that the body relies on *both* fat and carbs for energy all the time, albeit in different ratios. In fact, right now as you sit here reading, you may be burning about 50-60 percent fat and 50-40 percent carbohydrates. You're not using much of either, however, because the amount of calories you need probably amounts to about one or two calories a minute. If you were to get up and start jogging in place, your body would need to supply you with some quick energy to do so, so the metabolism ratio might shift to drawing upon more carbo-hydrates, say 70 percent, and less fat, say 30 percent. If you were to con-tinue jogging, then, in order to preserve the carbs (which can run out since you have limited stores in the body), your body would gradually shift its metabolism ratio again to say, 60 percent fat and 40 percent carbohydrates. From an energy efficient point of view, it pays to be fit. The endurance athlete would be able to make the shift sooner, and his fat-burning percentage might be 65-75 percent.

  However, in practical terms this is purely technotalk, and these ratios don't make a big difference when it comes to losing weight and decreas-ing your body fat. For the most part, athletes are often leaner not because they might rely on slightly more fat for fuel, but because they practice their sport two to three, or more, hours a day — this burns a lot of calories. If you had the time, energy, and fitness level to work out three hours a day, being overweight would probably not be an issue. To lose weight, you need to burn more calories than your body consumes and uses everyday. Exercise is one main way to burn a lot of calories. But when it comes to weight loss, what matters is how many calories you burn, not so much whether they are fat or carbohydrate calories.

- **Myth:** Exercise done at a low intensity, such as walking, is better at fat burning than other high-intensity activities, like running or cardio activities where you push yourself very hard.

  The Truth: In a strict scientific sense, these claims are true because working at a lower intensity requires less quick energy and a higher percentage of fat is burned. But you'll also burn fewer calories than you would if, for the same amount of time, you work out at a harder intensity (running versus walking). If you're trying to lose weight, even though a higher percentage of fat is being used, a lower total amount of fat is lost.

  Whether increased fat burning will result in actual weight loss is depen-dent upon several variables, including the total calories burned (which include both fat and carbohydrate calories) and the total fat calories burned. If you do work at a low intensity, you need to increase the time spent exercising to burn more calories. What matters most is the total number of calories burned. If you burned 250 kcal every day from a short, fast jog, you'd see a bigger difference in weight and fat loss than if you walked everyday for the same amount of time. The number of fat calories you burn isn't that important, because even if you burn a lot of carb calories, these need to be replaced both by the carbs you eat in your diet and also within your body. Your fat stores will be broken down and transformed into carbohydrates when you need fuel. Even if you're burning lots of carb calories and less fat calories through exercise, your fat still inevitably gets used.

It boils — not burns — down to this: During the same amount of time you don't use more calories at lower exercise intensities. If you're trying to lose weight and you have only 30 minutes to work out, you would burn less calories walking at a moderate pace compared to walking at a fast pace. Working out at higher intensities may cause you to burn a lower percentage of fat, but since you burn more total calories, you still use more fat calories.

Low- to moderate-intensity exercise can burn a significant number of calories over a period of time. If you aren't fit enough to push yourself to work at a high intensity, or you have a physical weakness that prevents you from doing so, you can still burn a lot of calories by doing low-intensity workouts for a longer period of time.

✔ **Myth:** Running, cycling, or other cardio activities are more fat burning once you've been doing them for more than 15 or 20 minutes.

The Truth: Technically, once you've been exercising for 15 or 20 minutes, your body has made the shift to using a higher percentage of fat for fuel. But again, if you're trying to lose weight, it's about the total number of calories burned, not necessarily the fuel source.

For example, let's say at rest you burn up to 60 percent fat. When you enter the initial phases of intense exercise, the ratio changes. You may now burn only 30 percent fat because your body is using quick-energy carbohydrates. Once the exercise is sustained, the body switches back to using a higher percentage of fat to fuel the movement (up to 75 percent fat). In this aerobic phase of exercise, a higher percentage of fat is being used for energy. But if you aren't working out for a very long period, you may still burn more total calories and, therefore, more fat calories working out harder. Put another way, if burning as many calories as you can is the best way to lose weight, even a dummy can figure out which activity of the following is going to give the best results (answer: jogging and sprinting), even though their fat-burning quota is on the low end of the ratio.

Activity	Calories Burned	Fat Percentage	Calories from Fat
Watching TV for 20 minutes	40 kcal	60 percent	24 kcal
Walking for 20 minutes	100 kcal	65 percent	65 kcal
Jogging & sprinting for 20 minutes	250 kcal	40 percent	100 kcal

Pulling the Pieces of the Fitness Puzzle Together

You may have heard fitness banter being tossed around: "I'm going to go do some cardio" or "That was an aerobic, not an anaerobic workout." The terms are enough to confuse even the fittest of folks, especially since some of them refer to the same thing (cardio and aerobic). So often the lingo is misinterpreted, leading to even more confusion. In this section, we introduce all the pieces of the fitness puzzle. You'll use these elements — cardio stamina, muscle strength, power, flexibility, and sports skills — to create a well-balanced exercise program.

Huff-n-puff: Cardio stamina

When you do an exercise that involves your whole body moving for an extended period of time, your heart and lungs have to work harder to get your blood pumping faster so that your body can produce the energy you need to be able to continue moving. This causes you to huff and puff (or at least breathe heavily). This type of exercise is *cardiopulmonary* (cardio=heart and pulmonary=lungs), or *cardio* for short.

Although you use your arms and legs, you tend to use many muscles at once. Unless you're just starting out or doing some activity at a very intense, very competitive level, you probably won't fatigue any one muscle group. You use many muscles at a low to medium intensity, and you perform the activity for an extended amount of time.

Aerobic exercise

Although your body uses some carbohydrates and other forms of quick energy for fuel, with this level and duration of movement, your body uses slightly more fat as an energy source. In scientific jargon, this is known as your *aerobic metabolism* — often this type of whole body activity is called *aerobic*. (Don't get this confused with *aerobics,* which refers to the group exercise or dance-based cardio classes where you do a series of moves such as kicks, jumping jacks, and knee lifts.) Aerobic exercise can include aerobics, but it also refers to walking, running, cycling, swimming, aerobic dance, stepping, and activities that you'd do on cardio machines like the stair-stepper, rower, or elliptical trainer.

To make things more confusing, aerobic exercise can also become *anaerobic* if you jack up the intensity because you shift your fat- and carbohydrate-burning ratios. And what's aerobic for some may be anaerobic for others, depending on each person's fitness level. The unfit person burns more carbs; the fitter person is more efficient at consuming energy so he burns more fat.

Anaerobic exercise

Anaerobic exercise refers to the physiological state where your body uses a higher percentage of carbohydrates for fuel (although it still also uses fat). Anaerobic exercise can refer to slower, isolated muscle activities like weight lifting and calisthenics exercises like push-ups. It can also be aerobic exercise that is performed at a higher intensity — sprinting versus jogging, for example. The distinction is a physiological one. At any given time, our bodies use an equal amount of fat and carbohydrates for fuel. When we ask our body to become more active and expend more energy, the body draws upon these two main fuel sources in different ways. If we need to suddenly run to catch a bus, our quickest source of energy is from the carbohydrates. If we need to go on a very long walk, the body will shift from using an equal ratio of both energy sources to using a higher percentage of fat the longer the exercise goes on.

Sometimes stop-and-start activities such as tennis, football, basketball, and soccer are said to be anaerobic. However, it is clear that they work your whole body, and the heart and lungs do a lot of work. In fact, determining whether a whole body activity is aerobic or anaerobic is really just a physiological distinction that you in your exercise life probably don't need to worry about. What matters is that you're moving and burning a lot of calories, plus strengthening your heart and lungs and developing stamina in the muscles you're using when you do whole body activities. Check out Chapter 6 for more details on cardio training.

Heave ho!: Muscle strength

Some people misuse the word *strong*; to them, saying that a part of your body is strong is just another way of saying physically fit. A runner, for example, may be said to have a strong body because he can run for long periods, but in the pure sense of the word, he actually may not be very strong.

The real definition of *strength* is the ability of a muscle or muscle group to produce force. The stronger you are, the better you can lift, push, or pull heavy things.

Strength is important when it comes to protecting and supporting your joints. All of the major muscles in the body surround different joints. Muscles absorb most of the load around the joints. If the muscles are strong, the joints have less stress. **Remember:** A strong muscle makes for a happy joint.

Unfortunately, our muscles don't get strong by themselves. They need a little push . . . well, actually a big push. Muscles become stronger when they are challenged to overcome more resistance than they are normally required to overcome.

All types of exercise — from walking to weight lifting — involve varying degrees of resistance. Low-resistance exercise may develop other aspects of physical fitness, but it won't make you strong. The more resistance your body has to overcome when it exercises, the stronger the muscles targeted will become. For example, when you walk, your leg and arm muscles can move pretty easily with each step and arm swing, so walking is a low-resistance exercise. If you walk uphill, through mud, or against wind, your muscles must work much harder against these different kinds of resistance to move and propel your body forward. Hill climbing is a higher resistance exercise than regular walking. Cycling in a low gear makes your legs have to exert much more force to pedal; swimming fast through water requires much more muscular force than if you were to do the same arm and leg movements in the air. Most cardio exercise offers low-to-medium resistance to the body. What is officially known as *resistance exercise* are exercises like push-ups, squats, biceps curls, and ab crunches where you move some sort of weight (even just your body weight). We answer your weight lifting questions in Chapter 14.

The long haul: Muscle endurance

Endurance is a muscle's capability to contract repeatedly over a period of time. The more muscular endurance you have, the longer you can last without getting tired. You develop muscular endurance by doing cardio activities — running, cycling, swimming, skating, and so on. Endurance and strength are complementary, but different, aspects of muscular fitness. Marathon runners, for example, have excellent endurance in their legs, however, they might not be very strong. Weight training also develops muscular endurance, although how you weight train (the number of repetitions you do, the speed, and the amount of weight you lift) determines to what extent.

One appealing result of training your muscles is that they become firm and more sculpted. You tend to get firmer and more sculpted from training for strength, not endurance. Many old-style fitness class exercises that "went for the burn" by doing lots of repetitions of exercises quickly focused on developing endurance, not strength, in the muscle. Now fitness classes have changed the way they condition. You're more likely to hear instructions to pick up weights, slow down the movements, and do only 12-15 repetitions at a time of a move because this is the best way to get strong and get firmer. Find out more about your muscles in Chapter 7.

Hang loose: Flexibility

A body can walk around tight and stiff, or it can move with freedom and suppleness. Some people take the joys of suppleness too far and develop too much flexibility. A joint is flexible if it can move freely in its natural range of motion. What that range of motion is depends on the joint. A knee joint, for example, works like a door hinge: it bends and straightens. It doesn't rotate, twist, or revolve like the ball-and-socket-style joint in the hip. If your knee can do more than just bend and straighten, you're too flexible. This can leave the joint unstable and increase your risk of injury. Some types of activities like yoga, gymnastics, and dance encourage extreme flexibility in order to attain some body positions. And as impressive as it might look to twist yourself into a pretzel, for most people, developing this range of flexibility is not desirable and can cause chronic joint damage.

Still, many people never bother to improve their flexibility at all and they grow stiffer with age. This can leave a joint too rigid, also increasing the risk of injury. Your best bet is to do activities that keep all parts of your body moving. Check out Chapters 15 and 28 for more details on safe stretching.

Flexibility involves increasing the suppleness of the muscles around a joint, as well as some of the other joint tissues, including tendons and cartilage. The easiest way to improve flexibility is by stretching.

Stretching isn't the only way to get flexible. Any type of exercise that requires you to bend an arm or leg or lean your torso in different directions will improve your flexibility. Studies show that even weight lifting can improve your flexibility. The important thing is to move your joints.

Pow! Zap! Bam!: Power

Muscle power is when you can exert a lot of force *quickly*. Most people don't focus on developing power as part of their fitness program unless they play sports. Many sports movements require that you push heavy bodies (football), carry your own heavy body across space as fast as you can (basketball, soccer), or hit fast objects coming to you with precision and speed (baseball, tennis). All of these actions require powerful muscles to execute them well. You can develop muscle power with exercises where you move quickly against some sort of resistance. This includes jumping, lifting weights quickly, sprinting, swinging a bat or racquet, and so on. We include special exercises to help you be more powerful in Chapter 20.

Sports skills (speed, agility, and coordination)

A fit body has good cardiovascular stamina, muscle strength, endurance, and flexibility. But a fit body can take fitness to a higher level by developing more challenging skills:

- *Speed* is the ability to move your body across space quickly, whether it's when running, cycling, swimming, or walking.

- *Agility* is the ability to move quickly and easily while stopping, starting, and turning. You need to be agile in most sports in order to respond to the different game situations where you have to dodge a ball, go after a ball, scoot away from an opposing team member, turn around and change directions, and so on.

- *Coordination* is the ability to do complex tasks, often involving simultaneous movement of the arms and legs. Coordination is something learned through practice and the result of your brain, muscles, and nerves working together in a programmed, synergistic way. A few examples include executing a series of dance or aerobics steps, or completing a tennis serve or basketball lay-up.

We include special drills in Chapter 21 to improve your speed, agility, and coordination.

Overload: The Secret to Getting Stronger

No one is born strong. We're born with the potential to make our bodies stronger (and we mean strong in the non-weight lifting sense here). We can create superhero bodies by improving all of the aspects of physical fitness — from cardio stamina, muscle strength, endurance, power, speed, agility, and coordination. The secret to doing that is *overload.*

As you exercise, your body becomes stronger. It also enables you to do increasing levels of exercise. You can do an aerobics class without getting as tired as you did when you first started. You can walk farther. You can lift more weights. In order to keep improving, the body must be subjected to controlled overload. That is, there must be a progressive increased stress on the muscles and system involved. If not, the body will respond by maintaining, but not improving, its current fitness level. Have you ever hit a plateau? You may have experienced results at first but after a while nothing more seemed to happen. It could have been that your body had successfully adapted to the challenge you gave it at first. When you ceased to keep challenging it, it ceased to keep adapting.

You can increase the overload by manipulating the frequency, intensity, or duration of your exercise. When you feel yourself completing each of your sessions very easily, mix things up:

- ✔ You may want to add another day per week.

- ✔ You can make your sessions last longer.

- ✔ You could push yourself harder — walk faster or concentrate on resisting with your arms more.

It's best to vary the ways in which you stress your body. For instance, suppose you decide to overload by increasing the duration of your workout by five minutes each week. If you start walking for 30 minutes, several months later you could be walking up to two hours a session. Obviously, this is impractical for most and would possibly cause you to drop out rather than continue. A better approach would be to walk a little longer on some days, walk a little faster on some days, travel over more hills on some days, and cycle on other days.

You have limits on your overload. If you try to increase at a drastic rate in order to get quick results, it can backfire. You cannot speed up certain bodily processes. Muscle conditioning, for example, requires that you allow 48 hours rest in between resistance training sessions so your muscles have time to heal and become stronger. In some cases, an elite athlete may recover more quickly than this and therefore be able to work the muscles more often. But most people need the full recovery time. If you push it and work the same muscle groups very intensely every day, rather than giving them a break, you may hurt yourself or at least hamper the rate of your improvements.

Fat loss, too, cannot be sped up. Every time you exercise for 30 minutes you may use 200-400 calories (depending upon what you do). Not until you have used several thousands of calories over a period of months will you see a noticeable difference in body shape from the *outside*. You simply can't hurry the process because it is virtually impossible to use up the calories any quicker.

Remember to overload *gradually* so your body has time to adapt to the changing stimuli before you increase the stress further. As you get older, your body takes longer to adapt, so you may want to go even more slowly than you used to.

Chapter 3

Variety Is the Spice of Life

In This Chapter

▶ Varying your workout five ways

▶ Rescheduling your hour of exercise

Cross-training is not sticking to the same old routine that you've grown to know and love. Cross-training is not about getting too comfortable with your current condition. Cross-training is not about being predictable. Doing the same workout all the time will not only bore you and leave you more prone to injuries, it can keep you from getting the results you want.

Cross-training is about adventure and trying new things. You don't have to be the adventurous type, though. It's not necessarily about trying bungee jumping, rappelling, or white water rafting. Cross-training is about making little changes to your present routine, so even if the only thing that's new is the angle of your biceps curl. Cross-training is the solution for everyone, whether you're a sometime exerciser that wants to look better or a competitive athlete whose aim is to develop advanced sports skills. This chapter shows how you can inject variety into your exercise life; we include daily, weekly, monthly, and yearly tips.

Five Ways to Vary Your Workouts

Here are five ways you can switch up and organize your workouts:

✔ **Switch to different activities:** Does the stair-stepper in the left corner of the gym have your name on it? Next time, head to the rowing machine. Sneak into a step class. Try something new.

✔ **Vary how you train:** If you walk regularly, some days you can walk slowly over a long distance, and other days you may want to alternate walking and jogging. Other days you may want to focus on walking a mile as fast as possible. You can also utilize items in the environment to get you working harder: If you see steps, walk up and down them, walk backwards and sideways, walk up hills, and so on.

✔ **Splice same-old, same-old workouts:** Instead of one long run, insert some stair climbing every time you run past a stairway. Or if you're in the park, do step-ups on every fifth park bench you see. Get off that stationary bike midway and run for five minutes on the treadmill.

✔ **Try different moves with different tools:** You don't have to use the same set of dumbbells all the time. A new wave of resistance equipment is flooding the gyms, giving you hundreds of more ways to do the same old exercises. Use stability balls, weighted medicine balls, exercise bands, balance boards, a step, barbells, weighted vests, and so on.

✔ **Up the ante:** Push yourself a little bit harder than usual: Run faster, increase the weight you lift or the number of sets you do, perform a more difficult version of an exercise, pair up exercises together to superset, or change the order of the exercises you do in a session.

Varying Your Daily Workouts

To give you an idea of all the different single session workouts you can do, we provide some routines that you can follow both in the gym and outside. As well as giving you a breakdown of time intervals (how many minutes to spend during each phase of a session), we include intensity levels to work at during each interval. You will see a number that corresponds to the Perceived Rate of Exertion scale in Chapter 6. Check out Chapter 6 for more information on how to gauge how hard you're working out. Remember to modify the intensity and time of any interval by either slowing down or speeding up, or shortening or lengthening a time slot as you feel fit.

The Cardio Machine Variety Hour

Recharge your machine routines with this cross-training approach to gym workouts. When you get on each machine, enter the time that you want to stay on that machine and then choose the manual mode in order to change your intensity level. Pick a time when the gym is less busy and move as quickly between machine stations as you can. Use as many different machines as possible. Substitute machines when necessary. Shorten the workout to 20-40 minutes if you're a beginner by shortening the length of time of each interval and/or using fewer machines.

10 minutes	Warm up on the bike.
5 minutes	Climb the revolving step machine (exertion level 4).
5 minutes	Walk on the treadmill (exertion level 4).
5 minutes	Walk uphill on the treadmill (exertion level 4, incline 1.0 grade).

5 minutes   Row on the rowing machine or rowing ergometer (exertion level 4).

10 minutes   Step on the stair-stepper (exertion level 5).

10 minutes   Ride on the elliptical trainer (exertion level 4).

5 minutes   Climb on the climbing machine (exertion level 3).

5 minutes   Cool down on the recumbent bike.

The Weight Circuit Variety Hour

Using free weights and cardio machines or different cardio options perform two exercises followed by a cardio interval. Try to allow no more than 30 seconds between sets. Substitute exercises and cardio options when necessary.

10 minutes   Warm up by walking on the treadmill; move arms in different directions slowly.

3 minutes   Perform two sets of squats (see Chapter 16).

3 minutes   Perform two sets of military presses overhead (see Chapter 17).

2 minutes   Step up and down on a bench (exertion level 3).

3 minutes   Perform two sets of plié squats (see Chapter 16).

3 minutes   Perform two sets of biceps curls (see Chapter 17).

2 minutes   Jog in place or on a treadmill (exertion level 3).

3 minutes   Perform two sets of back lunges (see Chapter 16).

3 minutes   Perform two sets of triceps kickbacks (see Chapter 17).

2 minutes   Do jumping jacks (exertion level 4).

3 minutes   Perform two sets of lunge scissor kicks (see Chapter 18).

3 minutes   Perform two sets of rubber band rows (see Chapter 17).

2 minutes   Jump rope (exertion level 4).

3 minutes   Do the walk-thru lunge (see Chapter 18).

3 minutes   Do push-ups (see Chapter 16).

2 minutes   Perform knee lifts in place or step on stair-stepper (exertion level 3).

10 minutes   Cool down by walking on the treadmill or marching in place.

The Running Variety Hour

Do this walk/jog/run workout on a treadmill or around your block. Shorten the more intense intervals as necessary.

15 minutes	Warm up by walking from a slow to brisk pace.
5 minutes	Jog (exertion level 3).
5 minutes	Jog faster (exertion level 4)
5 minutes	Jog slower (exertion level 3).
2 minutes	Run as fast as you can (exertion level 5).
5 minutes	Walk (exertion level 4).
2 minutes	Run as fast as you can (exertion level 5).
5 minutes	Walk (exertion level 4).
5 minutes	Jog (exertion level 4).
3 minutes	Pick up the pace and run (exertion level 5).
8 minutes	Cool down by walking.

The Playing Field Variety Hour

Here's a good cardio blast. All you need is a good pair of running or cross-training shoes and your local school ground. Decrease the time as needed.

10 minutes	Warm up by walking around the field.
10 minutes	Start from one corner and run to the diagonally opposite corner; walk down the side of the field to the opposite corner; then run to the diagonally opposite corner; repeat.
10 minutes	Move sideways along all four sides of the field doing the *carioca* — shuffle moving to the right by stepping out with the right foot and crossing the left in front, then stepping out with the right foot and crossing the left in back quickly. On each long side of the field, alternate the lead foot.
10 minutes	Move backward doing back lunges across the length of the field.
10 minutes	From diagonally opposite corners, run to the opposite corner lifting your knees as high as you can.
5 minutes	Do jumping jacks.
5 minutes	Cool down by walking around the field.

The Home Fitness Variety Hour

Bring out your dumbbells and/or rubber resistance bands and sneak this intense total-body workout into your day.

5 minutes	Warm up by walking around the block.
10 minutes	Run around the block.
10 minutes	Alternate 3 sets of 12 jumping jacks and squats (see Chapter 16).
10 minutes	Step up and down off a step or stair in your home.
10 minutes	Alternate 3 sets of 12 back lunges (see Chapter 16), push-ups (see Chapter 16), and biceps curls (see Chapter 17).
10 minutes	Alternate 3 sets of 12 rubber band rows (see Chapter 17) and lateral raises (see Chapter 17).
5 minutes	Cool down by marching in place.

Mixing It Up Weekly and Monthly

You've seen how you can mix things up within one session, but you should also keep the variety in throughout the week and from month to month. We suggest that you do at least two to four different activities per 12-week cycle of training, with at least two different activities per week.

The Cross-Training Plans in Part III add the freshness factor you need. You can keep the changes coming by following different plans; for example, start with the Base Fitness Plan, move on to the Weight Loss Plan, and then try the Athletic Plan. You can follow the weekly plans exactly, or you can switch the types of workouts you do around, as long as you stay within the recommended exercises guidelines. An example would be if you complete your cardio workouts on most days, but change your strength workouts around, making sure that you allow a day of recovery between strength workouts.

Keeping It Fresh All Year Long with Periodization

Athletes keep their bodies active all year long, but they can't keep the same level of fitness going all year long because their bodies need a break. That's where periodization comes in. With *periodization,* you mix things up by focusing on different aspects of fitness at different times of the year. You've probably heard of athletes being in off-season and in-season training. This is how they cross-train, and it's very specific. A coach may look at the athletes' fitness program over a year and organize it into periods of ever-changing workouts.

A *macrocycle* is the long-term plan. If you were a professional athlete, your macrocycle would be a length of time that includes your off-season and on-season. *Mesocycles* are the increments in between (the off-season or on-season). Then the day-to-day schedules that follow the formula needed for each mesocycle are *microcycles*. Any of these periods can be as long, or as short, as you plan. Generally, however, a training period, or mesocycle, that focuses on developing one particular aspect of fitness will be 6-12 weeks because this is the minimum amount of time it takes to see significant changes as a result of an exercise program.

Periodization is the most technical way to cross-train. It allows you to constantly vary your routine in a systematic way. You can focus on improving your strength by doing intense weight workouts for a few weeks. Then, you can lay off the supersets and go back to a minimal amount of weight work to maintain your gains while you focus on improving your running speed or throwing technique. You can then cut down the cardio frequency and return to more heavy-duty weight work, but focus on developing more explosive power, while still keeping up a low level of cardio work. This sort of on-and-off-again, mix-it-up approach is a great way to keep your body stimulated, which ensures good results, and will also help you vary the stresses you put on your body — a surefire way to keep your injury risk low.

While most of us aren't able to look at our workout in the long term, you can adopt the spirit of periodization by putting a little organization to your fitness planning. We make it easy with the plans in Part III. You can either pick one plan to do, or you can follow them in order for a long-term approach. Or you can just be aware that as you implement cross-training into your daily and weekly workouts, you'll want to vary your overall routines on a monthly or bimonthly basis as well by phasing in other kinds of workouts or changing the formula of your workouts.

How old are your shoes?

How long will your shoes last? Most podiatrists advise that you first try a change of shoes if you're experiencing foot problems from exercise. When shoes become worn out, they lose much of their cushioning and shock absorption. The general rule is to buy new shoes every 350-500 miles or after three months. Don't be fooled that just because you've been on an exercise hiatus for six months that your shoes will feel brand new. If they've been exposed to heat and sunlight, the material of the shoes can harden and decrease their shock-absorption capabilities.

Choose the shoes you use

In the early days of sports, athletes had very few shoes to choose — then emerged a shoe for every sport. In recent years, the cross-trainer has entered the spectrum, claiming to be the shoe you can wear for a variety of sports. So what's the lowdown? Are cross-trainers really enough? Or should your shoes be as specific as your workouts?

When it comes to styles, the shoe you choose can make a difference. The foot reacts differently in different sports. Laboratory equipment can measure the various impact forces, muscle activity, and the angles at which the foot lands during moves such as jumps, side steps, half and full turns, running, and so on. Plus, a greater understanding of foot biomechanics has helped improve shoe design. In theory, a sports-specific shoe will help correct and protect a foot from the stresses inherent in a particular sport.

For example, when you run, the impact force between the ground and your body is magnified. The foot lands in a heel-to-toe pattern. A running shoe should focus on minimizing some of the pounding force and provide stability at the heel since it's the first thing to touch the ground. Tennis, on the other hand, doesn't involve too much landing force but does involve lots of shuffling forward, backward, and sideways. The shoe needs to provide a stable base with lateral support for the multidirectional movement. Aerobics also involves traveling in many directions, as well as increased landing forces. As opposed to running, most of the steps in aerobics involve toe-to-heel landing. An aerobics shoe needs more cushioning at the ball of the foot, but it also needs to be stable to cope with the twists and turns.

Cross-trainers are built to be all-round shoes with a good degree of stability and shock absorption. They come in indoor and outdoor versions. If you're doing a random selection of activities, cross-trainers are a good shoe to choose. If you're serious about a particular activity and will spend more than one hour a week doing it, it's a good idea to invest in the appropriate shoe.

Cross-trainers will still work as an all-purpose shoe, but you may notice a big difference in how easily you move and how comfortable you feel if you try a shoe suited for your particular activity. Keep in mind, however, they're just shoes! While the improved materials and design of shoes today may help you reduce your risk of injures, even the best shoes can't make you run faster, play harder, or score the winning goal.

Part II
Let's Get Specific

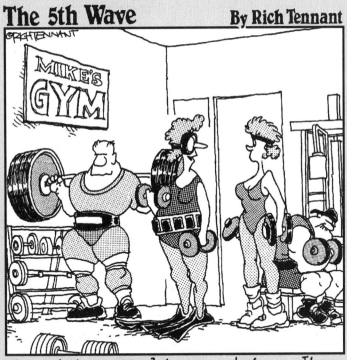

The 5th Wave By Rich Tennant

"I heard it was good to cross-train, so I'm mixing my weight training with scuba diving."

In this part . . .

You're going to take a good hard look at where you are in your fitness life and where you want to go. We show you why you need to have a specific destination in order to do the right kind of workouts that will get you there. Then we explain the smart way to plan your training. You'll test your fitness levels to find out where your body needs strengthening. You'll also consider the special factors about your body, your lifestyle, or your interests that may affect the type of workout program you'll do.

Chapter 4

Get A Goal
(Be Smart Before You Start)

. . . .

In This Chapter

▶ Setting your targets

▶ Utilizing the Fitness Formula

. . . .

To cross-train, you need to figure out what you want and what you need to do to get it. Some people exercise for the fun of it (we think there's not enough of these people). Some people work out for a flatter belly, impressive biceps or pecs, or thinner thighs. Some people like to win, so they train doing different competitive activities like running, cycling, or team sports. Some people like the way that exercise makes them feel — peaceful, less stressed, and revived. There are lots of reasons to exercise, but unless you turn them into concrete goals, you might be exercising on the path to nowhere. That's not to say that you won't experience the benefits of exercise during each and every workout. You just might not be working toward achieving anything specific. And if deep down you really do want serious results, you might not get them. In this chapter we help you pinpoint what it is you expect from your fitness routine.

Oh, the Possibilities . . .

Your first step in creating a fitness plan is to ask yourself, "What do I want to get out of my exercise routine?" Here are some examples of what's possible when you exercise. Exercise can

✔ Improve your overall health.

✔ Increase your energy levels.

✔ Give you a stronger butt, shapelier arms, sculpted thighs, and firmer abs.

✔ Improve your mental well-being and ability to handle stress.

✔ Rehabilitate you from an injury.

  ✔ Thwart some of the signs of aging, such as sagging, drooping, slowness, and fatigue.

  ✔ Improve your throw, kick, swing, and other sports skills.

  ✔ Give you an outlet to vent your feelings.

  ✔ Lower blood pressure and resting heart rate; increase the amount of blood that the heart pumps out per stroke, improving your cardiovascular efficiency; and improve other physiological things that make you feel better.

  ✔ Improve your posture.

Whether you experience any or all of these effects (or more) depends on your exercise prescription: what you do, how you do it, and how often you do it. In smaller, less intense doses, you'll improve your overall health, but that won't be enough to get you through a triathlon. If you exercise frequently but stick to mostly stretching and walking the dog, you're probably not going to change your body shape very much, nor will you develop the skills to play better tennis.

Setting Targets and Getting Specific

Once you have established the *reasons* why you want to work out, you need to define your *goals*. Making a *smart* goal — a Specific, Measurable, Attainable, Realistic, Timed goal — will set you on the right path to achieving it. Goals are tricky things. It's easiest to make a lofty, vague goal. If your goal is not *specific,* though, it's hard to define what it takes to get there. So rather than think, "I want to improve my tennis game," think, "I want to improve the accuracy of my serve."

Your goal should be specific enough to be *measurable*, that is, you should be able to tell when you've attained it. If you want to improve the accuracy of a serve that's mostly out of the court, you'll be able to tell when you've improved this skill — your serve will be placed in the forecourt for the majority of attempts.

Make sure that your goal is actually *attainable.* If you're aiming for aces, yet you've only just picked up a tennis racket, your goal may be beyond your abilities. It may take you hours of developing basic serving skills before you can start to perfect them. Shooting for something big is good because the higher your goal, the more you will achieve to attain it. Even if you don't ultimately reach this goal, you will have progressed further than you would have if you aimed for something lower. However, to achieve your big goal, you need to be *realistic* and determine the intermediate steps that will lead you to it. To prevent getting lost or bored along the way, you need to make a big goal smaller by figuring out how to achieve the baby steps you'll need to make to get there. If you make your goals unrealistic so that you don't get some sort of interim result to keep you motivated, you'll simply never reach your destination.

Finally, you need to make *timed* goals so that you have a beginning and end point. This will keep you focused and give you the leeway to modify your goal along the way. It's fine to take six months to lose five pounds, but if you were really expecting to lose it in six weeks, it's going to be hard to keep yourself motivated to stick to the workouts and healthy eating plan you need to do to lose it. Make sure your time-frame is realistic, though, and don't expect miracles overnight. Your body can change and will improve, but it takes time and commitment.

Big goal	*Baby steps to achieve goal*
"I'm going to lose 30 pounds."	"I'm going to lose 5 pounds in 8 weeks."
"I'm going to run a marathon."	"I'm going to run a 5K in September."
"I'm going to improve my health."	"I'm going to start incorporating 15 minutes of activity into my life every day (starting today), and then work up to 20 minutes in three weeks."

Now that you have your goals in mind, what do you need to know to achieve them? Bring to mind the main components of fitness (see Chapter 2 for a refresher): cardio stamina, muscular strength and endurance, flexibility, power, speed, agility, and coordination. Different types and amounts of exercise will help you develop each of these aspects of fitness. But for your workouts to give the results you want, you have to get specific and follow the Fitness Formula for your goal. (We explain what the Fitness Formula is in the next section.) If you're training for a sport and want to play better basketball, part of your Fitness Formula would entail developing running speed, improving cardio stamina, and practicing making baskets. If you're trying to improve your health or lose weight, you would get specific by making sure that the exercises and activities in your plan are the type that will give you those results. When exercising to improve your health, often all it takes is a little bit of low-intensity exercise. When trying to lose weight, you may need a formula that has you exercising harder and more often.

In many cases, the benefits of fitness are linked — train for cardio and you will automatically develop muscular endurance; train for speed and you'll automatically get cardio benefits, stress relief, and probably weight loss. However, if you want to improve your tennis serve, jogging won't do much — practicing the serve over and over and strengthening the muscles involved in serving will. It may be that you don't need to do as much as you think you do. Or, you may need to do more or something different.

Using the Fitness Formula to Reach Your Goals

The great thing about exercise is that we've had lots of smart exercise physiologists take the hard work out of working out. Research shows us how to be much more efficient by pinpointing the best ways to train. One of the results of all their sweating and toiling away in the human performance laboratories (yes, that's what they're called) is that we now have fairly accurate formulas outlining the exact fitness prescription it takes to elicit certain results.

The American College of Sports Medicine (ACSM) periodically assesses all the research that's been gathered and revises the generally accepted recommendations as needed. Most personal trainers, coaches, and physical therapists design their exercise plans base on these guidelines. We base the Cross-Training Plans in Part III on these general guidelines (see Table 4-1).

Table 4-1	Fitness Training Guidelines			
Type of Exercise	*Duration*	*Frequency*	*Intensity*	*Goal*
Cardio Stamina	20-60 minutes	At least 3 days a week	Moderate	To maintain current fitness level
Cardio Stamina	20-60 minutes	4 or more days a week	Moderate to high	To improve current fitness level
Cardio Stamina	20-60 minutes	4-6 days a week	Moderate to high	Weight loss
Muscle Strength	About 10 exercises	2-3 days a week	All major muscles	Strength
Flexibility	Hold each stretch for major muscles at least 10-60 seconds	2-3 days a week	Slow, static	Suppleness
Sports Skills	30 seconds to 2 minutes	1-2 days a week	High	Power, speed, or coordination

Periodization: Achieving goals without burnout

Although a new exerciser will generally experience positive changes no matter what he does or how he does it, as long as he is doing something productive, the regular exerciser can become stagnant and plateau if he does the same old thing for too long. *Periodization* is the ultimate training formula that can optimize your results. It's a way of mixing up things in your workouts so that you focus on different aspects of fitness at different times of the year. You've probably heard of athletes being in off-season and in-season training. This is how they cross-train, and it's very specific. A coach may look at the athletes' fitness program over a year and organize it into periods of ever-changing workouts. See Chapter 3 for more information about periodization.

We've used these general guidelines to create a number of Cross-Training Plans in Part III. All you need to do is pick the plan that will best help you reach your goal:

- **Base Fitness Plan:** Helps you develop a standard level of fitness with an emphasis on the basics: cardio, flexibility, and muscular strength. Chapter 9 introduces this plan.

- **Weight Loss Plan:** Helps you boost your metabolism to lose unwanted inches. Chapter 10 covers the Weight Loss Plan.

- **Athletic Plan:** Brings your base fitness to a higher level while honing in on developing the speed, agility, and coordination you'll need to excel at different sports skills. You can find the Athletic Plan in Chapter 11.

- **Mix-n-Match:** We also give you a template so you can custom-design your own plan for more specific goals. Chapter 12 has the format for a plan that you can devise yourself.

Although Table 4-1 includes the standard formulas you should follow when planning out your program, you do have some flexibility. For example, studies have shown that you can break a 30-minute session into three 10-minute sessions each day and still experience similar results.

Chapter 5

Weak? Who Me? Just Test Me!

In This Chapter
▶ Cross-training check-up
▶ Testing your fitness status

*B*efore you jump into your new cross-training program, you need to take yourself on a test drive. You wouldn't screech out of the used-car lot onto the freeway without a full assessment of the car's driving record and repair history. We don't expect you to break into an Olympic sprint and hurdle toward your fitness destination without taking a closer look at how your own nuts and bolts are holding up.

Exercise is good for you, but it can still be a stress to the body and exacerbate pre-existing weaknesses. So before you start any exercise program, get the go-ahead from your doctor. Even if you do have some limitations, chances are you can still exercise; you'll just have to modify what you do by doing less challenging exercises and less vigorous workouts to best suit your body. In this chapter, we put together a group of home tests so you can get an idea of what kind of shape you're in.

Testing, Testing

Fitness tests can be elaborate or simple. The more medical versions, like the maximal stress test, where you're plopped on a treadmill wired up to electrodes and gas masks and asked to run as hard as you possibly can, are used to gauge such scientific aspects of your fitness as your maximal oxygen consumption and metabolic rate. These sorts of tests are done under expert supervision at sports medicine clinics, hospitals, or university human performance labs. Modified versions of these tests, which give you estimates of your fitness health, are often given at health clubs as part of the initial screening process and for periodic progress evaluations. We like Chapter 2 in *Fitness For Dummies,* 2nd Edition, by Suzanne Schlosberg and Liz Neporent (IDG Books Worldwide, Inc.), which gives a good breakdown of all the standard tests and what they mean, plus some you can do by yourself. Before you begin any exercise program or do any home fitness tests, get a doctor's approval.

Cross-Training Check-Up

We've put together a series of self-tests that you can use to give you a general idea of your strengths and weakness. Once you know what areas need to be addressed, you can incorporate your results into your Cross-Training Plans in Part III to help navigate your plan to focus on the areas you need to work on most. After 8-12 weeks, you can do another check-up to see how you've improved from your starting point. You can then switch your fitness emphasis in your next cross-training cycle based on your results.

The following exercises gauge your cardio stamina, muscular strength, endurance, speed, agility, balance, flexibility, posture, power, and body shape. ***Remember:*** These are only tests, only estimates, and only to be used as a rough guide to chart your progress. Don't get too hung up on the results because lots of variables can influence how you perform. Unless you have a fitness professional overseeing as you perform these tests, your results won't be accurate enough to make sweeping assumptions about how fit (or unfit) you are. Even the standard tests in health clubs have flaws. The ratings about your level of fitness on various tests are usually based on estimates from studies done on subjects that may be nothing like you, say, Swedish, 19-year-old male phys ed students. Your 25- or 45-year-old sedentary body with a totally different bone structure than the average 6'6" tall Swede may score differently simply because you're different, not because you're less fit. The flexibility test is a perfect example: If you try to touch your toes, the person with longer arms and shorter legs will score the best every time, but that's not an indicator that he's as flexible as he should be.

Martica knows of a model who had a fitness evaluation at the health club she belonged to. Although the girl was 5'10," weighed 125 pounds, and was clearly too thin for her own good, the gym instructor who tested her reported that her body fat was 30% (technically her levels categorized her as medically obese). This discouraged the poor girl so much that she quit working out. Not only did the tester probably perform the test incorrectly, some common sense needs to be applied to the outcome. Sure, the model probably was lacking in muscle mass, which upped her body fat percentage, but obese she was not and to suggest she lower her body fat, rather than build up muscle and increase her weight, was probably a dangerous recommendation.

How to start: You can try some of them or all of them. Each body check we include is meant to assess the different components of fitness that you will improve as the result of a cross-training program. Check your status now, and then reassess in 8-12 weeks. After following one of the Cross-Training Plans in Part III, you should notice a major improvement in how you perform these exercises.

Try not to exercise before taking these tests. Wear comfortable clothes and if anything hurts during any tests, stop and skip it. Place your answers in Table 5-1 as you go along. When you get to the body measurements section, enter your answers in the spaces provided. Then transfer the total amount to Table 5-1.

Table 5-1	Home Fitness Evaluation Worksheet		
Starting Date: _____			
Body Check Test	*First Measurement*	*8-Week Measurement*	*12-Week Measurement*
Heart			
#1: Resting heart rate			
#2: Exercise heart rate			
#3: One-minute recovery heart rate			
Flexibility			
#4: Flexibility			
Stamina			
#5: Stamina			
Posture			
#6: Deep ab strength			
#7: Spinal alignment			
#8: Back slump			
Agility			
#9: Jump power			
#10: Upper body power			
Speed			
#11: Sprint speed			
Core Strength and Endurance			
#12: Core strength			
#13: Core endurance			
#14: Hip stability			

(continued)

Table 5-1 *(continued)*

Starting Date: _____

Body Check Test	First Measurement	8-Week Measurement	12-Week Measurement
Control			
#15: Dynamic movement			
#16: Static balance			
Body Fat			
#17: Body Mass Index			
#18: Waist-to-Hip ratio			
#19: Upper body measurements total			
#20: Lower body measurements total			

Heart

Do you get winded after one flight of stairs? Is what stops you from exercising longer the fact that you're out of breath, rather than your muscles getting tired? The fitter you are, the lower your pulse will be in the morning when you wake up and the quicker your heart gets back to its normal heart rate after a bout of exercise. This test counts your heart rate in beats per minute (bpm) during these two conditions.

Body check 1: Resting heart rate

When you first wake up, before you even get out of bed, place two fingers (not your thumb — it has a pulse) on your wrist below the base of your thumb. Count the beats in 15 seconds. Multiply this by four for the number of heartbeats per minute.

Body check 2: Exercise heart rate

You will step up and down off a step for three minutes. You'll need to control the speed at which you step, so pick music with an even dance beat, but it shouldn't be too fast. Start by facing the base of a step, bench, or stable chair (6-18 inches high). Step up with your right foot firmly in the middle of the platform (don't allow your heel to hang off the back edge) and then step up with your left on top of the step. Step down with your right and down with your left. Repeat this foot pattern. Stop after three minutes and immediately feel your pulse and count the number of beats for one minute, not by using a heart rate monitor, but by taking it yourself.

Body check 3: One-Minute Recovery heart rate

After this minute, take your pulse again. Note your one-minute recovery heart rate, either by counting or using a heart rate monitor

When you do this test again, make sure you use the same step and same music to ensure that you replicate the way you performed the test the first time.

What it means: Generally, the lower your resting and post-exercise heart rates are the more efficient your heart is (it pumps less to get the same amount of blood through the body). An athlete may have a resting heart rate of 40-60 bpm; the average healthy person is usually 60-70 bpm. (But remember that medication, stress, or any exertion in the hour or two prior to taking your heart rate can elevate it.) Vigorous activity can elevate you to up to 180 bpm. Since fitter hearts recover more quickly from exertion, a post-exercise heart rate of 90-120 bpm is ideal.

Flexibility

Our bodies grow stiffer with age. Although any exercise, including weight lifting, will improve your flexibility and range of motion, it's important to include bonafide stretching sessions dedicated to relaxing and lengthening your muscles into your weekly workouts. Although every muscle is different, here's a test to get an idea of how flexible, or inflexible, your hamstrings in the back of your thighs are.

Body check 4: Flexibility

Measure a 12-inch length of tape. Place it on the floor perpendicular to a tape measure or yardstick so it intersects at the 15-inch mark. Sit with your legs extended. Your feet should face the tape. Straddle the tape measure with your legs, and place the zero mark toward your crotch. Lean forward without bouncing for one minute to relax your muscles. Then stretch your arms straight toward your feet to see how far your hands can reach. Read the number on the tape measure. See Figure 5-1 for an illustration of how this test should look.

What it means: Unless you have extraordinarily long arms, this move indicates the flexibility of your hamstrings (back thighs) and lower back. Aim for a reaching score of 16-19 inches or more. But remember, this only tests one area of your body. You may be more or less flexible in other muscle groups.

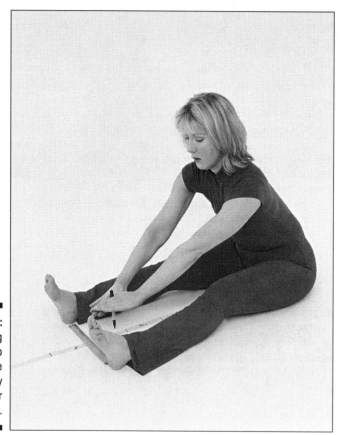

Figure 5-1:
Use a leg
stretch to
measure the
flexibility
in your
hamstrings.

Stamina

Your lasting power is an important aspect of all cardio workouts. Stamina is a mixture of heart strength and breathing power, with a little muscle endurance thrown in. One of the first signs of being out-of-shape is early fatigue. However, once you start working out, it's one of the first improvements you'll notice.

Body check 5: Stamina

Chart a one-mile course outside. (Measure the distance in your car, or find an athletic track — four laps usually make a mile.) Warm up by walking briskly for 10 minutes. Then time how fast you can run or walk the course. (If you feel dizzy, stop.)

What it means: If you can walk the distance in 12 minutes or less, you have reasonable cardio fitness. Of course it can always be improved — a world class runner can do it in under four minutes!

Posture

How you hold yourself is a 24-hour occupation. Your spine should retain its natural S-shaped curve so that all your other body parts stack evenly into place. Your spinal alignment and the balance of your shoulders, ribs, and hips doesn't only affect the way you look when sitting or standing, it affects the way you move. As muscles weaken with age and inactivity, your posture will go along with them. Sticking to a regular exercise program, especially when you concentrate on maintaining perfect posture throughout all the training you do, will have long-lasting effects on your posture even when you're not working out.

Body check 6: Deep ab strength

Stand sideways in front of a mirror. Lengthen your spine by lifting your rib cage away from your pelvis so that you stand as tall as you can. Focus on the layer of abdominal muscle below your bellybutton; inhale and poof it out as if you were pretending to be pregnant. Then exhale and pull in these muscles to flatten the area from hip to hip to pubic bone.

What it means: This exercise targets your deepest layer of abdominal muscle, the transverse abdominis. If you're unable to successfully flatten your lower ab area by contracting this muscle group, the muscle may be weak. The transverse is a key muscle for postural stability. When you run, walk, dance, stand, and so on, it helps keep your hips still and support the lower back.

Body check 7: Spinal alignment

Hang a weighted string or rope from the top of a doorway. Stand behind it in a profile view so that it falls next to your ear. Stand with your feet hip-width apart. Hang your arms by your sides in a normal standing position, as if you were waiting in line at the grocery store. Ask a friend to monitor your body alignment, or take a picture (front and side view) so you can check yourself. Figure 5-2 shows an example of slumped posture, and Figure 5-3 shows good body alignment.

What it means: Looking at your profile, your ear should be above your shoulder; your shoulders should be underneath, not in front of, your neck. Looking at your front view: Your shoulders and hips should be parallel, not lopsided. Both shoulders and hips should be even.

Figure 5-2:
One example of a misaligned spine (side view).

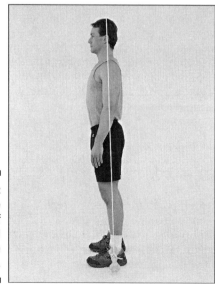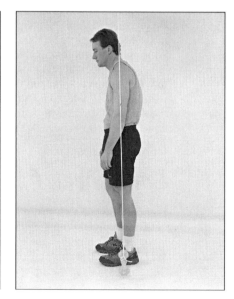

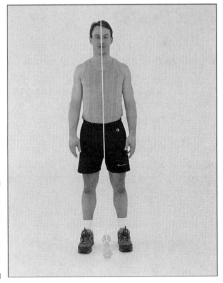 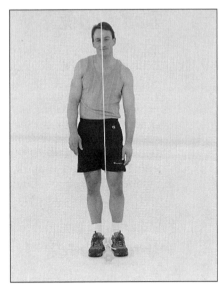

Figure 5-3:
Listen to
your mother.
Stand up
straight!

Body check 8: Upper back slump

Sit on a hard chair or stool in your normal relaxed sitting position. Have a
friend monitor you or take a picture, or sit in front of a mirror and take a
sneak peak at your posture.

What it means: Is your chin in front of your shoulders? Is your upper back
slumped? Does your spine have a C-shape, rounded curve? Is your chest
sunken in between your shoulders? Ideally, you should hold your rib cage
high, lower your shoulders and pull them slightly back, push your chest forward, straighten your spine or slightly arch the lower back, lengthen the
neck, erect your head above the shoulders, and tuck in your chin.

Agility

Lightness on your feet will enable you to exercise with ease — whether
you're scrambling over rocks on a hike, or dodging opponents during a football game.

Body check 9: Jump power

Stand with your profile next to a wall. Hold a piece of chalk, a pencil, or a loop of inverted scotch tape on your middle finger. With your feet hip-width apart, arms hanging by your sides, lower your body slightly by bending the knees, and then swing your arms and spring up. Jump, touching the highest point you reach on the wall with your inside arm. Mark the spot with the chalk, pencil, or tape. (See Figure 5-4 for an example.)

What it means: Repeat this jump three times. Measure the height you jumped from the floor to the mark, noting your score each time. Average the three numbers. This score should improve as you start getting fitter, especially if you incorporate some of the power moves in Chapter 20 into your routines.

Body check 10: Upper body power

Lie face down on the floor. Place your hands just outside your shoulders, palms down, fingers forward. Curl your feet under so your toes push against the floor. Push your body up into a lifted prone position. Drop your hips so that your entire body is in a straight line. Inhale and bend your elbows to lower your chest to the ground. Exhale and straighten your arms to push back up. Avoid moving your hips up and down to simulate the push-up movement. Perform as many push-ups as you can in one minute with good form. If you're not up to supporting all of your body weight, lower onto your knees, but keep the torso in a straight line throughout. Some women who have never completed a push-up this way may find this difficult. Make note of your number so that you can assess your improvements from regular stength training.

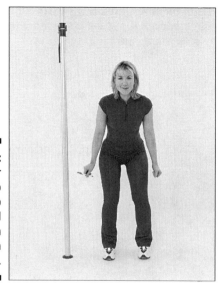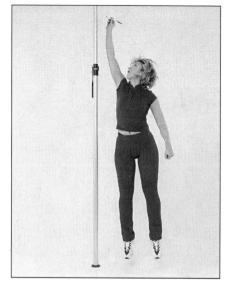

Figure 5-4:
Lower your body to spring up (left) and jump as high as you can (right).

Speed

When it comes to most competitive activities, how fast you move is crucial to getting ahead. Speed is an advanced skill and this test should only be attempted if you have been exercising regularly and have developed a good base level of fitness.

Body check 11: Sprint speed

Mark out a 40-yard distance on a track, or along a street or park path. First warm up for 10-15 minutes by walking briskly. Then, using a stopwatch, or having a friend time you, run as fast as you can along your 40-yard distance. Repeat twice and pick your best score.

What it means: As your body develops cardiovascular stamina, strength and muscular endurance, you are able to subject yourself to higher levels of intensity. Muscle fibers learn to contract at a faster rate, and you improve the fitness of your fast twitch, or explosive fibers. Make note of your time so you can see improvements later. Remember that although speed is a learned skill, the bigger, taller and heavier you are may also affect how fast you go.

Core Strength and Endurance

Your quality of movement and ability to control your body during all activities and exercises depend largely on the strength of your 'core', or muscles in your middle. It's not just about rippled abs, but functional abs that help support your spine, along with all the other muscles in the back and torso.

Body check 12: Core strength

Start on your hands and knees. Place your hands slightly wider than shoulder width; keep your palms flat and fingers pointing forward. Extend both legs behind you, and balance your body weight on your toes and hands. Drop your hips so that your shoulders, hips, and ankles are in line (see Figure 5-5). Maintain a regular breathing pattern, and time the number of seconds you can hold this position before your abs, back, and other muscles in the torso fatigue. If your wrists feel uncomfortable, lower yourself onto your bent elbows and forearms.

What it means: If you can hold your body in this position for 1-2 minutes, your torso muscles are in good shape. If you can only hold yourself up for 15 seconds or less, concentrate on utilizing your abdominals during all the exercises that you do.

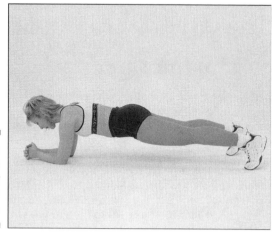

Figure 5-5:
Balance with your body in a straight line.

Body check 13: Core endurance

Lie on your back with your knees bent, feet flat on the floor, arms straight by your sides, and hands on the outer sides of your legs. Tighten your lower abs to move your rib cage forward, closer to your hips. Reach your arms out by your sides. Lower your shoulder blades to the floor. Repeat as many ab curls as you can in one minute (see Figure 5-6).

What it means: This move requires endurance of the abdominal muscles. If you can do 45 curls within a minute, your muscles are in good shape. If you can manage less than 20, focus on engaging the abs during all the exercises that you do.

Body check 14: Hip stability

Lie on your right side, and hold both arms straight down in front of and close to your body. Rest your head on the floor, and then raise your left hip toward the ceiling to arch your body so that you're balancing on your shoulders and outer right ankles. Hold for as long as you can in a stable balanced side lift.

What it means: If you can hold your body up for more than 15 seconds, it's a sign that your gluteal muscles in the hips are strong. These muscles are important for overall stability during movement.

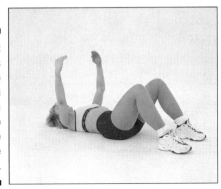 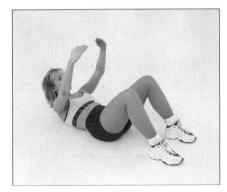

Figure 5-6: Complete as many ab curls as you can in a minute to test the endurance in your abs.

Control

Fitness is not just about strong muscles, but it is about strong muscles that work well in sync with each other. Once your body is strong enough to hold itself in a variety of positions, you can challenge it to maintain control in more dynamic, unbalanced movements.

Body check 15: Dynamic movement

Stand with your feet together, hip-width apart. Lunge your right leg back. At the same time, bring your right arm up in front, left arm straight by your side in the back. As you squeeze your left glute and hamstring to straighten, raise your right leg up in front of your body and kick your foot forward (keep it below hip level) as your right arm swings back and left arm swings front (see Figure 5-7). Lower and repeat. Do as many kicks as you can in one minute with control.

What it means: If you can do 20 kicks in one minute, you have excellent control and stability. If you can do less than 10, concentrate on incorporating balancing movements within your strength exercises. You can follow the multimuscle movements in Chapter 18 to see your improvement soar.

Body check 16: Static balance

Stand with both feet hip-width apart, and place your hands on your hips. Raise your right leg in front. Keep it straight and lift slowly up as high as you can without tilting your pelvis or losing balance. Spread the toes for a stable base of support in your standing leg. Avoid letting your upper body slump; hold your ribs high throughout. Hold for as long as you can.

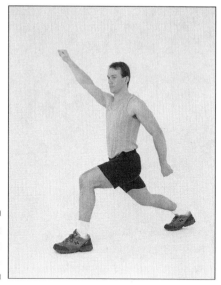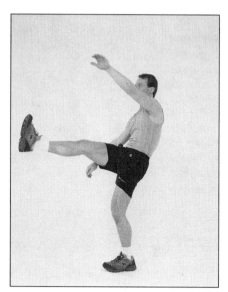

Figure 5-7:
Kick with
control.

What it means: If you can hold this position for 60 seconds, your balance is very good. If you can only hold this position for less than 15 seconds, concentrate on moving slowly through all the standing strength exercises that you do to develop better control.

Body Fat

How good you look in your fitness gear and everyday clothes is more dependent upon your body fat and muscle tone than your weight on the scale. Plus the amount of body fat you have, and where you carry it, can indicate your susceptibility to serious illness. However, be aware that you can be fat and fit! So don't get too hung up on those last few pounds that might be biologically very difficult for you to lose. If weight and fat loss are your goals, you'll want to include these tests to gauge your progress.

Body check 17: Body Mass Index

You'll need a calculator for this one. Divide your weight in kilograms (1kg=2.2lbs) by the square of your height in meters (1 meter=39.4 inches) to determine your Body Mass Index (BMI).

What it means: Body Mass Index predicts overall health, but if you're fit and muscular, or very thin and unfit, you might get an inaccurate reading. Those with a BMI of 20-25 live the longest. Over 30 indicates obesity and a greater risk of serious diseases.

Body check 18: Waist-to-Hip Ratio

Then divide your waist measurement by your hip measurement to determine your Waist-to-Hip ratio.

What it means: Women should aim for a ratio below .8, and men should aim for a ratio below 1.0.

Body check 19: Upper Body Measurements

Using a cloth or paper tape measure, measure the circumference of your body at the widest part of the following sites. (Figure 5-8 shows you the precise locations for taking body measurements.) Mark down each number, and then add the numbers for the upper body to reach a total upper body figure.

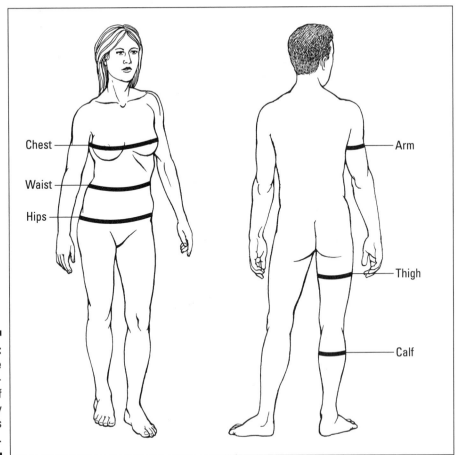

Figure 5-8:
Measure
the circum-
ference of
the body
part at its
widest area.

Chest

Waist

Hips

Arm

Thigh

Calf

Table 5-2	Upper Body Measurements		
Starting Date: _____			
Body Part	*First Measurement*	*8-Week Measurement*	*12-Week Measurement*
Widest part of upper right arm			
Chest			
Upper rib cage			
Waist			
Abdomen (around bellybutton)			
Total upper body			

Body check 20: Lower body measurements

Using a cloth or paper tape measure, measure the circumference of your body at the widest part of the following sites. Mark down each figure, and then total the number for the lower body measurements.

Table 5-3	Lower Body Measurements		
Starting Date: _____			
Body Part	*First Measurement*	*8-Week Measurement*	*12-Week Measurement*
Widest part of hips (around buttocks, below hip bones)			
Upper right thigh (widest part of thigh)			
Mid right thigh			
Above knee, right thigh			
Right calf (widest part)			
Right ankle			
Total lower body			

What it means: Everybody has different sites of body fat. By getting as specific as possible when measuring your body, you can detect changes in areas that you might not otherwise have noticed (above the knees, rib cage, and so on).

Your Results . . . and What They Mean

So you've discovered that you can barely do one push-up, your back hurts when you try to do too many ab curls, and you wobble like crazy when you try to balance. On the other hand, you could run faster than you expected and your jump isn't so bad either. What do you do with this knowledge?

No matter what strengths and weaknesses you may have, it's important to first approach every exercise and activity with caution, especially when a movement looks like it may put your weak areas under excess strain. If you have joint problems, high-impact activities, such as running long distances and using heavy weights, are probably not the best type of exercise for your body. If you have difficulty balancing, you're better off doing slow, simple moves rather than faster, more complicated ones. If you found that you are fairly strong but get out of breath from doing the stamina test, you may want to focus on building up your cardio stamina before improving your strength.

Parts IV and V give a wide range of exercises and activities that you can include in your Cross-Training Plan. However, not all the moves and activities are right for every body. When you perform the exercises, make sure you follow the instructions exactly and pay attention to how your body feels as you do the movement. (Chapter 13 shows you how to use your mind to enhance the way your body moves.) When choosing cardio activities or sports, take it slowly. We include suggestions on how to improve your performance in these areas in Part VI.

Chapter 6

Huffin' and Puffin' Cardio

Cardio workouts are activities that get your whole body moving for an extended period of time. Your heart and lungs work harder to get your blood pumping faster so that your body can produce the extra energy you need. What determines whether you feel pooped or ready for more is your intensity — how hard you push yourself during your workouts.

Your exercise intensity is also a predictor of the kind of results you'll see. The lower your intensity, the less overload there is on your body, and the less it is forced to make dramatic changes. The higher your exercise intensity, the more your body pushes itself — and the fitter, stronger, faster, and firmer you'll get because of it. Of course, the trade-off is the harder you work, the more unpleasant it can feel if you're not up for it. You also risk yourself with higher injury and drop-out rates with harder exercise sessions. So before you rush out for a ten-mile run, consider that most fitness experts purposely slow you down so that you'll still be around to exercise in a month. Working at a lower intensity is often the smarter way to train when it comes to sticking to it. However, sometimes you do have to push yourself to achieve the desired training effect. In this chapter we show you the workout intensities right for you and we help you gauge your intensity.

Measuring Your Intensity

You walk up a hill, and you huff and puff. You sprint for the bus and your heart beats double-time. You lift weights and feel like you don't sweat at all, yet one power yoga class makes you sweat bullets. How can you tell how hard you're working during all the different activities you do? You have several ways, from measuring your heart rate to monitoring your self-perceived sensations of how tired you feel as you exercise. Once you get used to a workout, it's easier to get a better innate sense of your intensity, and you can use these methods to work at different levels. Beginners often don't have enough familiarity with how their body feels during exercise to accurately gauge their exertion, so monitoring it throughout is a useful way to keep the workout safe and effective.

Calculating your heart rate

You can monitor your exercise intensity in many ways. You can estimate how hard you're working out based on your oxygen consumption — how much oxygen your body is sucking in to sustain you — by taking your heart rate. With every heartbeat, your body draws in more oxygen and circulates more blood around. The faster your heart beats, the faster your breathing gets to draw in more air and deliver more oxygen to the muscles that need them. Taking your heart rate is one way to estimate how hard you're working.

Check the pulse at your wrist, neck, temple, or heart for 6, 10, or 15 seconds. (Place any finger — except your thumb, which has its own pulse — on the site and then count the number of beats starting at zero within the number of seconds. Multiply by 10, 6, or 4 to get the number of beats per minute.) The resulting heart rate gives you an idea of what level of intensity you're working based on your maximum heart rate.

Your maximum heart rate varies with your age. The most scientific way to determine it is to take a maximal exertion test while strapped up to a heart rate monitor. These tests are always performed under the supervision of an allied health professional (a doctor, nurse, and so on). In theory, if you can reach the point where you're running or cycling as hard as you possibly can, just before your heart literally can't beat any faster, you could determine how fast your heart is able to beat. Since this is a pretty unpleasant and risky test, a guesstimate is made with a formula that subtracts your age from 220. So it can be assumed that the maximum heart rate of a 40 year old is roughly 180 beats per minute (bpm). You determine your exercise intensity, or different levels of exertion during workouts, based on your maximum heart rate.

To figure out what your exercise intensity is while exercising very hard, say, at 75 percent of your maximum, you'd multiply .75 by 180 bpm if you're 40 years old. Exercising at a heart rate of 135 bpm would then put you in the zone of working out at a high intensity. If you were to work out at a low-to-moderate intensity, then your exercising heart rate would be around 105, or 60 percent of your maximum.

This method isn't fool-proof, though, because many factors can influence how fast your heart beats whether you're exercising or not. You can be sitting in a chair and worried about how much work you have to do, and the stress could cause your heart to speed up, even though you're not actually moving. While you're walking, you could make arm movements overhead. This could raise your heart rate but in reality not raise your exercise intensity by very much. Some medications, including the caffeine in a cup of coffee, can speed up your heart rate artificially. Also, it can be difficult to count your pulse correctly during some activities, such as when you have lots of equipment that may get in the way. An exercise such as swimming can lower your pulse because of the cool water and horizontal position of the body. Cardio workouts that involve a lot of overhead arm movements can elevate the heart rate but not the intensity. Keep in mind that every body and heart are different. Estimating your heart rate is not an exact science, so don't worry if you're working out at a higher or lower heart rate, especially if you feel fine during the exercise.

Heart rate monitors are an easier way to see instantly how hard you're working. Many brands are available, most of which use a chest strap that takes your pulse and sends the signal to a wristwatch. You can see your heart rate change just by checking your watch. Many cardio machines have heart rate monitors too.

Taking the talk test

You can also take the talk test: If you can talk with little difficulty during your workout, you're probably at a lower intensity. If you're panting and can barely spit out a few words, you're working at a high intensity.

Gauging your perceived exertion

The easiest way to assess how you feel at any given moment during exercise is to ask yourself how you feel. This method, called the Perceived Rate of Exertion, is more accurate than you might think.

In the 1960s, Gunnar Borg, Ph.D., a Swedish exercise physiologist, developed a way to estimate exertion based on the perception of the effort level. He found that a direct link existed between levels of perceived effort and various heart rates. Through a numbered scale he designated certain feelings to indicate the level of the exercisers' exertion.

He began with the Level 0, representing effort that felt very, very light. The numbers at the higher end of his scale reflect exercising at an intensity that felt very hard. Borg found that even though his subjects were all of different fitness levels, if they all felt like they were working somewhat hard, they were all working at the same level of difficulty according to their personal fitness level. The scale numbers correspond to each individual's appropriate heart rate, or exercise intensity. (This method is much more accurate if you're a regular exerciser because you're likely to be more familiar with how it feels to exercise at different levels.)

During different points in your workout, select a number on the scale that reflects how you feel (see Table 6-1 for the scale). Focus on your overall effort, not on one sensation, such as how tired your calf muscles are. You can consciously raise or lower how hard you're working accordingly. General guidelines recommend that you aim to work at an intensity that you feel is somewhat hard (Level 4). This corresponds to working out at an intensity that is 65-70 percent of your maximum heart rate.

Table 6-1	Perceived Rate of Exertion Scale
Rating	**Description of How You Feel**
0	No exertion
0.5	Very, very light (just noticeable) exertion
1.0	Very light exertion
2	Light (weak) exertion
3	Moderate exertion
4	Somewhat hard exertion
5	Heavy (strong) exertion
6	
7	Very heavy exertion
8	
9	
10	Very, very heavy (almost max) exertion

Watch your breath

Another way to assess your workout intensity is by using the simple breathing scale developed by Michelle Scharff-Olson, Ph.D. Because your breathing rate increases (you take more breaths per minute) and your breathing volume increases (you breathe in more air per breath) during exercise, you can learn to become more aware of your intensity by focusing on how you are breathing. Check Table 6-2 below and notice whether your breaths are fast, gasping, short, deep, and so on. You can couple this information up with either your heart rate or Perceived Rate of Exertion to establish a better understanding of how your body feels during different levels of effort.

Table 6-2	Olson Breating Scale
Rating	*Description of How You Are Breathing*
1	
2	Very light
3	
4	Fairly light
5	Moderate
6	Moderately heavy
7	
8	Heavy
9	Very heavy
10	

How Hard Should You Exercise?

You're probably wondering how hard should you exercise. The rule is that there is no rule. It all depends on your goal.

A *target heart rate* falls between a range of about 50-85 percent of your heart rate max. Research shows that working at this level of intensity is enough to elicit physiological improvements in your cardiovascular health. It is sometimes said that you should stay in the low- to mid-point of the zone, between 60-65 percent, in order to get the most fat burning. But we know now that that's not exactly true. When it comes to fat burning, how many calories you burn overall is what matters, so you can burn a significant amount by either a longer workout done at a low to medium intensity, or a shorter workout done at a high intensity. Research shows that you can experience health benefits from very low levels of intensity. Working at higher levels can significantly improve your cardio stamina and other aspects of performance as long as you're fit enough to do so.

One method of working out called *heart rate training, zone training,* or *interval training* pushes you into different levels of intensity. Studies have found that you can work out harder and longer by breaking up a workout into harder "work" intervals and easier "recovery" intervals. So, you might exercise by alternating an intensity level of 7 on the Borg scale for two minutes, with slowing down to an effort level of 4 for five minutes. For the average workout, aim to work somewhat hard during most of your exercise session.

High or Low Impact: How Much Can You Take?

Compare a high jump with a long, fast run. Both are difficult and both stress your body in different ways. The jump is a high impact move — you need lots of explosive power in your muscles to execute it and your joints will feel a lot of pressure when you land. Compared to walking, the run is also high impact — your joints may feel up to six times your body weight with each step. But assuming your body is fit enough to carry itself, it's the speed that tires you out because your heart and lungs have to work at a higher intensity to sustain the movement.

Impact refers to the amount of force on your joints:

- ✔ *High-impact* activities include those that use pounding or fast movements in which both feet leave the ground temporarily. Jumping, running, and high impact aerobics are high impact activities.

- ✔ *Low-impact* activities have less landing force because you keep one foot on the ground, or your body weight is supported by something other than your feet during the activity (swimming, cycling, a stair machine).

Intensity refers to how hard you push yourself during a workout. High-impact activities are usually high intensity too. But low-impact activities can be performed at either a high or low intensity. Walking fast or uphill can be high intensity. If you push your heart to work in the upper ranges of your target heart rate zone, you are said to be working at a high intensity. You can work at a high intensity during easier activities simply by pushing yourself to move faster or adding some sort of resistance. Activities with more impact are often, by definition, a higher intensity because it takes more effort to deal with the impact. Both high-impact and high-intensity workouts are safe for many people, but it's important to realize the difference because you'll want to vary them within your overall training plan.

When Your Body Talks, Listen

Your body likes to send you signals in the form of aches, pains, and other sensitive spots of feeling *something* here and there. The beginning exerciser is usually quick to listen (looking for any excuse to quit), while the experienced exerciser is likely to shoosh the messages away, thinking it's something that can be ignored. Don't be fooled. You won't gain if you feel pain.

Pain is usually a sign that the body is being overstressed and perhaps damaged in some way. It can happen early on, as an indicator that something about the exercise isn't right. Or it can happen late in the game, when you've been overloading so much that eventually that tendon, ligament, or other body tissue has to give way to the stress. If exercise hurts, you should stop.

But this is where it gets confusing. Some exercise *does* hurt — like when you're lifting the last rep of the last set of arm raises. Or you're struggling to push the speed up that last minute of your run. So how can you tell the difference between good pain and bad pain? You'll find out in this section.

Feel the burn

Exercise can target a specific body part or muscle group and tire it out. A burning sensation in your muscles is a sign of depleting energy stores and waste buildup. When muscles contract repeatedly, lactic acid accumulates, and waste products build up faster than they are being carried away. When it's a cardio activity like running, this inhibits oxygen from being delivered to the working muscles.

We can group this burning sensation into two groups:

- ✔ **You're targeting a certain body part:** When you feel a burning sensation in the particular muscle you're working (when you're doing leg lifts, for example), providing that it stops when you stop the exercise, this is normal muscular fatigue. If you're doing weight training or exercises that target specific muscles, the muscle burning is an indication that you have reached a point of fatigue. Rest, and then do another set in a couple of minutes when some of the energy stores have been replenished.

- ✔ **You're working out your whole body aerobically:** If you're doing endurance exercise such as walking, swimming, or stepping and you feel burning in your muscles, you should stop or decrease the level of your activity. Since the aim of endurance, or aerobic activities, is to work all the muscles at once without fatiguing any one group, one group getting tired is a sign that you're working at too high an intensity.

Pooped out

Feeling dog tired? This could be a sign of a lack of sleep. You could be pushing too hard, be dehydrated, or be depleting your carbohydrate energy stores. Overall fatigue or weakness is not necessarily immediately dangerous, but you should slow down and rest because you are most prone to injuries when fatigued. Eat well and drink water before, during, and after your workout. You may also feel fatigued if you are overstressed or overexercising. Allow yourself to relax.

Owww!

Pain is a big red flag. If you feel discomfort in a specific area of your body, even a dull ache, you need to stop or modify how you're exercising immediately. Call your doctor if you feel it during times when you're not exercising. A minor pain can turn into an acute or chronic injury if you let it go for too long. Certain types of exercise — especially cardio — are meant to be fairly effortless. When you run or cycle, you're not purposely trying to fatigue a certain muscle group (as you might during weight lifting). So if you feel a specific site of pain in your back, thigh, or knee, something's wrong. If you're working at the appropriate level of intensity, a specific muscle group shouldn't respond with fatigue. Stop exercising immediately.

If you twist your ankle or incur a slight injury while you're exercising, don't ignore it; treat it right away. If you develop an injury, with your doctor's approval you don't necessarily have to quit exercising as long as you find a substitute that doesn't aggravate it. For example, instead of running on a sore foot, swim. If your injury prevents you from exerting much effort, meditate or take a walk. Keep up the active lifestyle even if you have to lessen the activity.

Tender to the touch

No matter what shape you're in, moving your body in a new way — especially if the exercise is strenuous — usually leads to some sort of post-exercise muscle soreness up to a day or two afterwards. If you're so sore you have difficulty doing *anything* the next day, you overloaded too much. Take it easy during your next few workouts. If you're *continually* sore, you probably aren't allowing enough recovery time in between workouts.

Poor performance

Sometimes your body gives you signs outside of exercise. You might be religiously doing your six-mile run, seven days a week, but if your body feels that you're working out too much, you might have these symptoms:

✔ Difficulty sleeping.

✔ Moodiness.

✔ Decreased appetite. (You might feel less hungry even though you're using up enough calories to require more, not less, fuel.)

✔ Constantly fatigued. (When you wake up in the morning you feel exhausted, or when you finish a workout, you feel tired, not revived.)

Overexercising leads to an impaired immune system — you may get chronic colds — and it can make you more susceptible to injuries. Remember that your rest days are as important as your exercise days. If you have any of these symptoms, allow more recovery time in between workouts and make sure you're getting enough sleep.

Do's and Don'ts of Cardio

Here are a few do's and don'ts to keep in mind:

- ✔ Don't sit if you can stand, don't stand if you can walk, and don't walk if you can run — push yourself to use your body as much as you can within your own safe limits.

- ✔ Vary your speed. To prevent your body getting used to the same workout all the time, go slow and long on some days, short and fast on others.

- ✔ Vary your zones. Pick different heart rates or numbers on the Perceived Rate of Exertion scale and work out at different levels during different sessions.

- ✔ Try interval training. Increase your intensity in bursts. Run, walk, or ride at a steady pace for 20 minutes, and then pick a lamppost (or time yourself) and work out harder for 1 minute. Slow down the pace and perform more energy bursts at random. Gradually increase the duration and frequency of your bursts to increase your overall intensity.

- ✔ Pick new activities. Try different sports and types of cardio workouts so that you continually force your muscles to adapt to new movement patterns.

- ✔ If you feel too winded, or if anything hurts, stop.

All about sweat

Sweat losses can vary from person to person. Some people hardly lose a drop, while others almost need to grab a mop to wipe up the pools of sweat from the floor. Sweating is the body's way to cool down its core temperature. The good news is that the more fit you become, the better of a sweater you become.

Exercise is hard work and high intensity workouts produce large amounts of heat. Bet you didn't know that death can occur if the body temperature is elevated only a few degrees above normal. So why aren't we all dropping off like flies?

Lucky for us, our body has a system of checks and balances that keeps the heat under control. During your workout, as your body heats up, the skin temperatures rises, the moisture leaving your pores evaporates, helping to cool the body.

This happens all the time, but we don't notice because the body is heated and cooled at the same rate so the sweat is not detectable. But during strenuous exercise, the body heats faster than it's able to cool off, which results in too much water loss to evaporate. So, the water beads off into sweat and pours off the skin. If you're sweating this much, you're not doing a good job of cooling off your body and instead you are dehydrating yourself.

Sweating without replacing fluid is not a good thing, either. The body contains over 60 percent water. Two-thirds of it is inside the cells and the rest is between the cells and in the blood plasma, the fluid portion of the blood. Water is vital to energy. If you become dehydrated, these distributions get imbalanced — you'll feel fatigued long before your glycogen stores run out.

Chapter 7

Gruntin' and Groanin': Muscle Strength, Stamina, Power, and Flexibility

*W*e don't walk around like robots because our muscles allow us to move in finely coordinated patterns. Without them we would collapse in one big heap of bones. Muscles are the support system that connects and moves our bones. They also give extra padding around the joints to make the body more durable. So often we fail to appreciate just how much precision and control we can move with.

Muscles come in different shapes and sizes. In this chapter, you'll get more familiar with what your muscles look and feel like and how they move. Some muscles are underneath others so it may be harder to isolate and identify the deeper ones. It's important to understand how your muscles work so that you can exercise with better technique. Plus, you'll know to include a well-rounded group of exercises and activities to ensure that your muscles are well balanced — equally strong and flexible throughout your body.

Gaining Total Muscle Fitness

Your cross-training plan should incorporate a range of activities that develops the following aspects of total muscle fitness:

✔ **Strength** is the amount of force a muscle can produce. Lifting progressively heavier weights helps you develop strength. The stronger you are, the better you can lift, push, or pull heavy things.

✔ **Endurance** is a muscle's ability to contract repeatedly or to keep an activity up for a long period of time before getting tired. You develop muscular endurance by doing cardio activities — running, cycling, swimming, skating, and so on — as well as doing higher repetition exercises with weights.

✔ **Power** is the ability to exert a large amount of force very quickly. A powerful movement may be as simple as jumping over a log as you walk in the park. For athletic endeavors, powerful movements are much more intense. To develop real power, you must train at a very high intensity. This can include doing speed work such as running, swimming, or cycling sprints. Or it can include doing jump training like plyometrics, where you make your body do explosive movements. Since only competitive athletes have a practical need for power, the average fitness plan won't include this type of high-end training. We include some power moves in some of the Cross-Training Plans (see Chapter 11 for the Athletic Plan if you're interested). *Remember:* These moves are high risk because they are so intense, and you need to have built up a good level of fitness before including them in your program.

✔ **Flexibility** is the range of motion a joint can move through. To be flexible, your muscles and other connective tissue around a joint need to be supple. You can improve flexibility simply by doing any type of exercise. You can hone in on specific areas by stretching different muscle groups. We talk more about the importance of flexibility in the "Adding Flexibility for Muscle Balance" section later in the chapter.

Meeting Your Muscles

Although you may have heard of muscle fibers, no one talks much about muscle cells. That's because a muscle fiber *is* a muscle cell. Whereas most cells in the body are microscopic, muscle cells are not. Muscles can be very big and so can their cells. Instead of the typical round cell shape, a muscle cell is a long cylinder that can run the length of the muscle. Some muscles, such as those in the eyes, may have just a few fibers. Big muscles, such as those in the legs, can have thousands of fibers. The more fibers a muscle has, the more force it can exert. Men tend to be stronger than women because they tend to have more muscle mass and therefore can exert more force with the same or less effort.

Moving your muscles

When you call a muscle into action, it produces force by shortening, or *contracting,* the muscle fibers involved. To do this, your brain first determines how hard a muscle must work. If you were to look at a bowling ball and a feather, for example, the brain assumes that one is lighter than the other and sends a signal indicating how many muscle fibers you need through nerves attached to the muscles involved in picking up the items.

A *motor unit* is a nerve and all its attached muscle fibers bundled together. One motor unit can have just two or three, a couple of hundred, or even several thousand muscle fibers. Another membrane encloses many muscle bundles, or motor units, to form the muscle. When your muscle contracts, some or all the fibers within the different bundles contract, depending upon the direction of the movement and how much force you need. When the brain sends a signal through a nerve, all the muscle fibers attached to that nerve contract 100 percent. However, most muscles have many nerves and therefore many different motor units. Not every movement activates all motor units in a muscle. To lift the bowling ball, for example, your brain activates the number of motor units needed for each specific action. A message is sent to the muscles that allow you to grasp the ball with your fingers; another message is sent to the muscles that contract the biceps so that you can produce just enough force to lift the ball.

For the best results during your workout, try to get as much muscle as possible involved by working as many motor units as you can. Perform the same exercise in different positions to activate different areas of a muscle. Vary the amount and type of force required by using different amounts of resistance, varying the speed of your exercises, and coupling up exercises together or manipulating how many reps and sets you do. By fatiguing your target muscle groups in different ways, you keep your muscles challenged, which helps them improve.

Introducing the two types of muscle fibers

Your body has two main types of muscle fibers, slow twitch and fast twitch (so-named because they contract at different speeds):

- ✔ *Fast-twitch muscles* are active during quick and powerful movements (for example, sprinting, jumping, or lifting heavy weights).

- ✔ *Slow-twitch muscles* have a greater endurance capacity and come into play during longer-lasting movements, such as jogging or lifting light weights.

Some muscles have more of one type than the other, especially if the muscles are designed for specific functions. The upper arms often have to pick up or push away heavy objects; they react with speed, so they are mostly fast twitch. Calves, which are a key postural muscle that needs to support a standing or walking body for long periods, are mostly slow twitch. In general, most muscles — and most bodies — are made up of a 50/50 split between fast- and slow-twitch fibers.

Then, there are those lucky genetic mutants. When they say that an athlete is born and not made, it's because some bodies have genetic predispositions toward certain physical attributes that can help them excel at certain sports. Just as a 6'6" basketball player has the edge over a 5'6" player, some bodies have an overall prevalent muscle fiber type that makes them better able to do well with certain types of movement, whether it's by being more powerful or having more stamina. A speed-sprint swimmer may have up to 80 percent fast twitch, while a long-distance cyclist or marathon runner may have up to 80 percent slow twitch.

You can tell if you're more inclined to one type over another by looking at the activities that you do well in. When you jog, do you feel better going long, slow distances? Or do you prefer to run fast and get it over with? Do you prefer basketball or softball? Slow-twitch types tend to have more staying power during sports, but generally do better at a low intensity. Fast-twitch types are quick, agile, and fast, but they tire out sooner.

Just as muscle won't turn into fat, you can't convert fast-twitch fibers into slow-twitch fibers, or vice versa. Research shows that with intense athletic and weight training some fibers may adopt characteristics of their opposite type, but they won't fully convert. That's why it's important to vary how you train so that you can target both types of fibers for total muscle fitness.

Pushing with your prime movers

Many people don't realize that you can train your muscles in several different ways. That's why one type of training, or one exercise, won't cut it when it comes to developing all-around fitness. You need to cross-train. Just because you have strong arms doesn't mean they have the stamina to swim long distances. A runner may have incredible endurance in his legs, but this doesn't mean that he is strong or able to jump powerfully.

How you work out determines how your muscles will adapt — they can grow stronger, develop more lasting power, or perform more explosive movements. Basically, they fall into two main categories: prime movers and stabilizers. The *prime mover* is the main muscle that initiates a specific movement. Your quadriceps, for example, are the prime movers in straightening a bent leg. Muscles can also assist or stabilize while other prime movers are working. For example, your abdominals and gluteals stabilize the torso during walking and running.

Strength Training to Get the Look

The beauty of muscles is that you can literally make them look better simply by exercising them. When a muscle gets strong, it gets firm and shows off its curves.

Challenging muscles to get stronger

When you work out hard, you challenge the muscle to exert as much force as it can. In doing so, the fibers break down, causing microtears. After stimulating the muscle, the muscle begins to adapt to the forces that stimulated it. Within approximately 48 hours of rest, the muscle fibers heal and grow stronger. This turnover process happens continuously. The other tissues surrounding a joint — including tendons that connect the muscle to the bones and ligaments that connect bones to each other — also become stronger when exposed to resistance. After a period of regular training, you become stronger from the rebuilding of the microtears and you fatigue more slowly, so you last longer.

What happens during this healing process changes during the course of your weight training:

✔ When you first start lifting weights, the muscle gets stronger — not by getting bigger — but by improving the communication and coordination between the brain, nerves, and muscle cells. This happens because your muscle learns to recruit more motor units, the coordination of how the motor units fire together improves, and the frequency in which the motor units contract increases. The more conditioned you are, the more quickly you'll be able to recover from one contraction and do another.

✔ After about 12-15 weeks of regular training, the strength improvements you see are no longer from these types of neurological changes but from the addition of more protein into the muscle fibers. The second stage is the *hypertrophy stage,* where your muscles, to a limit, can increase in firmness, hardness, and size as more protein packs into the cells.

Defining your muscles

How you work your muscles determines what they look like. When you train for strength, you often can change the size, look, and feel of a muscle. The stronger you are, the more *toned* the muscle fibers become. This means you'll feel firmer. If you're doing only cardio training, you probably won't get a hard body, especially in those muscles that don't do much work (the arms of a runner, for example). The firmer you want to be, the more you need to do specific exercises with resistance (weights or elastic bands, for example).

The stronger your muscle gets, the more defined it will look. You'll see its curves and sinews, providing, of course, that you don't have too much body fat on top of the muscle hiding its shape. Muscle definition is harder to achieve because it depends on your body fat levels. The more lean you are and the less fat you have, the more sculpted or *cut* your muscles will appear because less fat is filling out the curves of your muscles in your body. Combining calorie-burning exercise such as walking, aerobics, or cycling with your weight training will help you look more defined.

Muscles can increase in size only slightly. How big you get is largely genetic. Some people may be born with more muscle cells than others, so they might look more muscular. Your skeletal structure also plays a role. If you have shorter bones, you may look more muscular.

But no matter how hard you work, only half of 1 percent of the *male* population has the potential to develop the vein-popping bulges of a bodybuilder. Even people who want to look like Mr. Universe have to spend hours and hours lifting heavy weights and often taking steroids and other substances to look that way. Since women tend to have even less muscle mass and less testosterone, it's very rare for a woman to transform into a hulk. Plus, a little known secret about bodybuilders is they are not actually that big. They often diet themselves to extremely low — and often unhealthy — levels of body fat so that every muscle becomes visible. Prior to weight lifting competitions, they even eliminate salt and excess water from their body so they can look even more defined. If you're a casual weight user lifting 2-3 times per week, you'll have a very tough — if not impossible — time trying to look this way.

Adding Flexibility and Strength for Muscle Balance

Because the muscles' function is to provide stability and support for our skeleton, their overall alignment is a complex balance of tension and flexibility. If one side of the body is weaker than another side, postural imbalances leading to serious injuries can result. You must consider two aspects of balance in your training program: strength and flexibility. Each muscle group needs to have both.

Muscles generally work in opposing pairs: When a muscle group on one side of a bone contracts, the opposite side lengthens. An imbalance between the two can limit a joint's range of motion. When you bend your elbow, the biceps contract and the triceps lengthen in order for the arm to bend fully. If the triceps aren't very flexible, and the biceps are extra strong, strain and possible injury could occur from one forceful contraction. When part of the quadriceps contracts or shortens, it causes the entire lower leg to straighten at the knee. When this muscle group relaxes, the hamstrings in the back of the thigh contract, while the fibers in the quads lengthen so you can bend your knee.

Although several surrounding muscles may work simultaneously to perform a movement, most often the strongest one does most of the work. This can prevent the weaker ones from toughening up. While this can happen without you being aware of it — if you play tennis and use a one-handed backhand, or serve from the same arm, it can often be due to choosing an imbalanced group of exercises. It's easier to stick to your favorite moves exercising the stronger muscles since working out a weaker muscle can be hard work. But if weaker muscles aren't strengthened along with others in the body, the stronger ones could end up compensating for the weaker ones. This can lead to misalignments or excess strain on surrounding joints.

Another example is the shoulder blades. Most arm movements involve the shoulder blades in the upper back. More than eight different muscles move the shoulder blades up and down, forward and backward, toward or away from the spine, and so on. If one of these muscles is weak, the shoulder blades could be slightly off-kilter. This not only affects your ability to perform certain movements, it could also lead to postural and spinal problems.

Strong, well-balanced muscles protect the joints. For example, one of the biggest muscle groups in the body is the quadriceps — four muscles on the front thigh that join together to form attachments on each end. When your quadriceps are strong, they provide excellent protection for the knee joint. They help hold your kneecap in place. If you were to be kicked, or fall and twist this area, a strong muscle could help give you stability to resist the strain, or at least minimize the intensity of the injury.

The easiest way to make sure you are developing well-balanced muscles is to work all the muscle groups and vary your exercises periodically. It's also important to work in a full range of motion and call as many fibers in a muscle to work as possible.

Map Your Muscles

Look at each of the following muscle diagrams so that you can become familiar with your muscles. (See Figures 7-1 and 7-2.) Read the description and contract the muscle so you can feel it working. You can tell which direction a muscle will contract by looking at where it is attached and looking at the line of the muscle fibers. (Most anatomical drawings will lightly sketch these in.) So if a muscle attached to your spine has fibers that run horizontal to your body, you know this muscle will rotate the spine. Some muscles have fibers that run in several directions. This means that a portion of the muscle may be used during certain actions. When you train these muscles, it's a good idea to vary the exercises you do and the angles you work at so you target as much of the muscle as possible.

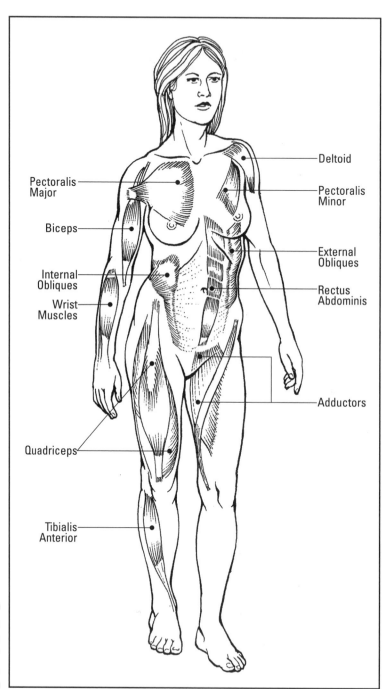

Pectoralis
Major

Biceps

Internal
Obliques

Wrist
Muscles

Quadriceps

Tibialis
Anterior

Deltoid

Pectoralis
Minor

External
Obliques

Rectus
Abdominis

Adductors

Figure 7-1:
A front view
of your
muscles.

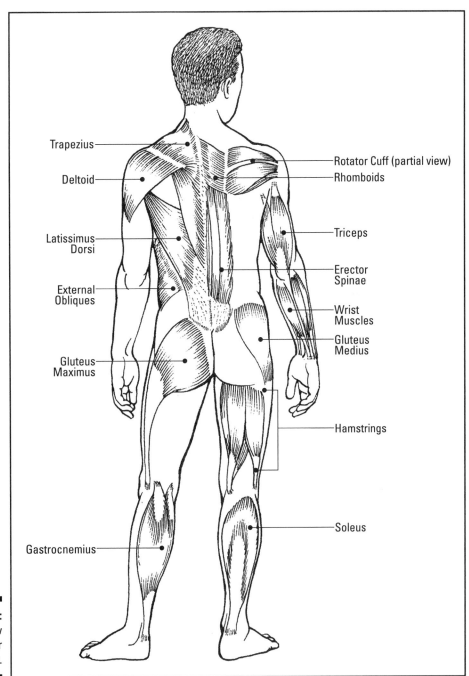

Figure 7-2:
A back view
of your
muscles.

A *concentric contraction* is when a muscle shortens to move the bones it is attached to in a particular direction. The same muscle then remains slightly contracted as the bones move back to their original position. This is known as the *eccentric* phase of the contraction.

Upper back

The *trapezius* is a triangular-shaped muscle on most of your upper back. (See Figure 7-3.) It covers most of your back, so you can feel it in several different places. Place your right hand on your left shoulder in between your neck and the rounded part of your shoulder. Lift your left arm to the side. Then place your hand on your back underneath your armpits and reach your hands out to the side and pull it back it. Finally, place your hand on the lower part of your rib cage on your back and reach up. This muscle contracts whenever you raise your arms and bring them back toward your body. It holds your shoulder blades in place.

The *rhomboids* are between your shoulder blades. Reach behind your back and place the back of your hand in between your shoulder blades on your upper spine. Now lift your elbows out to the sides keeping them shoulder level, and then pull your arms back behind you. These muscles contract and move the shoulder blades toward and away from each other.

The *latissimus dorsi* covers a very large area of your back. Reach underneath your arm and place your hand flat on top of the back ribs. Reach your hand out in front of you and pull the elbow back in to your ribs. This muscle contracts whenever you stretch out and pull in toward the body.

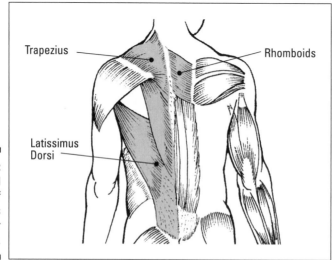

Figure 7-3:
Several layers of muscles cover your back.

Lower back

The *quadratus lumborum* is in the lower back, but is deep and difficult to feel. Place your fingers along the outer edge of your spine in the lower back. While your back is straight, press your fingertips deep into the muscle. Then bend to the side and back up to feel this muscle contract.

The *erector spinae* is along both sides of your spine from top to bottom (see Figure 7-4). Place your hand on the middle or lower spine and slowly bend forward, then straighten back up to an erect position. These muscles contract when your spine bends and straightens to all directions. They also play a large role in stabilizing your back for perfect posture.

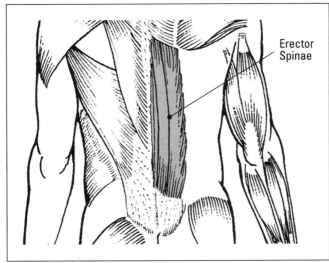

Erector Spinae

Figure 7-4: The erector spinae muscles support your spine.

Chest

Your *pectorals* are connected to your upper arm and breastbone (see Figure 7-5). Place your hand on the junction on the front side of your underarm where your shoulder and torso meet. Move your arm across your chest toward the opposite shoulder.

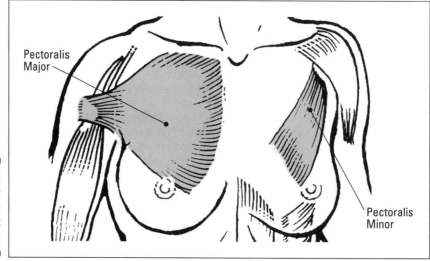

Figure 7-5:
Your
"pecs" are
your chest
muscles.

Shoulders

The *deltoids* are directly on top of your shoulder and when they are well developed they give you a nice rounded shape like a shoulder pad (see Figure 7-6). Cup your hand on the edge of the shoulder and then lift your arm directly up in front of you to feel the anterior deltoids, out to the side to feel the medial deltoids, and then up behind you to feel the rear deltoids. You can feel different parts of the muscle initiating the movement in each direction. This muscle raises your arm in different directions when it contracts.

Rotator cuff is a small group of muscles that are in and around the shoulder joint that help the arm rotate, such as when you're throwing a ball or hitting a tennis ball.

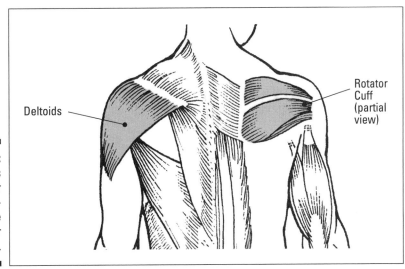

Deltoids

Rotator
Cuff
(partial
view)

Figure 7-6:
The deltoids
and rotator
cuff mus-
cles pad the
shoulder
area.

Arms

Triceps are in the back of your upper arms (see Figure 7-7). Place your hand
on the back of your arm, then bend and straighten your arm. This contracts
when you straighten your arm.

The *biceps brachii, brachioradialis,* and *brachialis* are in the front of your
upper arm. Place your hand on the front of your arm and bend and straighten
your arm. Hold it flexed — Popeye-style — and turn your wrist in different
directions to feel how different joint angles activate different parts of the
muscle. These muscles contract when you bring your hand to your shoulder.

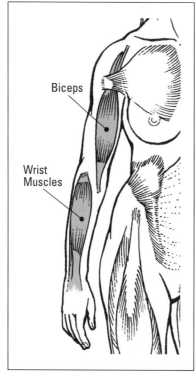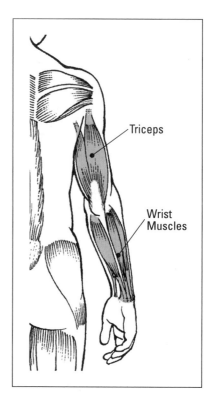

Figure 7-7:
Your arm
muscles
perform
highly
specific
movements.

Wrist flexors/extensors, which initiate wrist action, are in the front and back of your forearm. Grasp around the middle of your forearm and move your wrist back and forth. Notice the muscles on top tightening as your hand bends back, and then notice the muscles underneath the forearm contract as your hand drops forward.

Abdominals

The rippled-looking muscle that runs along the front of your torso from your ribs to your pubic bone is the *rectus abdominus* (see Figure 7-8). Lie on your back and place one hand just above and the other hand just below your bellybutton. Now lift your shoulder off the ground to feel the muscle contract. Notice how the contraction is stronger in the upper part. Next, bring your knees to your chest and tilt your pelvis forward. Notice that again, the whole muscle is contracting, but the lower end is working more.

The deepest abdominal muscle is the *transversus abdominis*. Place your hand flat on your lower abdomen. Make a cough or quick exhaling sound to feel this muscle pull the abdominal contents in.

The *internal and external obliques* run diagonally in both directions from your hips to the opposite ribs. Lie on your back and place one hand on the right side of your lower rib cage. Place the other hand just above the left hip bone and press in slightly. Now bring your right shoulder toward your left hip to feel the muscles contract.

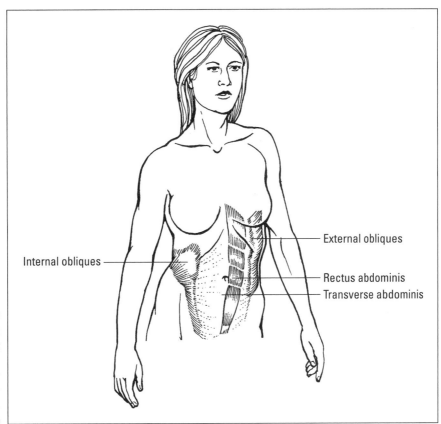

External obliques

Internal obliques

Rectus abdominis

Transverse abdominis

Figure 7-8: Get that "six-pack" look by working the abdominals.

Lower leg

The *gastrocnemius* is the rounded muscle at the top of your calf (see Figure 7-9). While standing, reach down and place your hand on the back of your lower leg. Lift your body weight on your toes so that your heel rises to feel this muscle contract.

The *soleus* is in the front of your gastrocnemius. In the same position as above, place your hand lower on your calf, just above your ankle. Lift your heel up and down to feel the muscle contract.

You can find the *anterior tibialis* in front of your soleus. You can feel it fatigue if you lift your toe to flex your foot repeatedly.

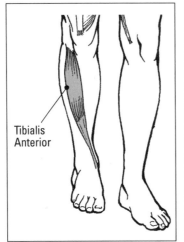 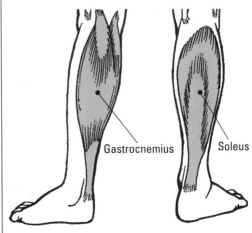

Tibialis Anterior

Gastrocnemius

Soleus

Figure 7-9:
The muscles of the lower leg.

Thigh and butt

The hamstrings (see Figure 7-10) consist of three muscles in the back of your thighs: the biceps femoris, the semitendinosus, and the semimembranosus. Stand up and place your hand on the back of your upper leg, and then bend your knee and lift your heel to your buttocks to feel these muscles contract.

The *quadriceps femoris,* or quads, are four muscles in the front of your thigh: the rectus femoris, the vastus medialis, the lateralis, and the intermedius. Place your hand on the front of your thigh. Bend and straighten your knee, and then lift and lower your thigh to feel these muscles contract.

The *tensor fascia latae* runs from the hip to just above the knee. Lie on your back. Place your hand on the outer hip between the hip bone and upper thigh. Then, lift your leg while turning it in to feel the muscle contract.

Five muscles in the inner thigh: the pectineus, the gracilis, the adductor brevis, longus, and magnus create the *adductor group*. Place your hand on the inside of your upper leg. Then lift your thigh and move it across to your opposite hip to feel these muscles contract.

The *hip flexors,* which consist of the iliopsoas and sartorius, are in the front of your thigh joining your upper leg and pelvis. Place your thumb on the crease between your upper thigh and pelvis. Lift your knee and thigh up toward your chest. You will notice two separate muscles. The one on the outside is the sartorius; the other is the top of your quadriceps (thigh muscles). The iliopsoas are deeper within the pelvis.

The *glutes* group (gluteus medius, minimus, and maximus) gives the buttocks a nice rounded shape. Stand up and place your hands on your bottom. Tilt your pelvis forward and back. Then, lift your leg to the side and to the back. Finally, bend your knees as if you were about to sit in a chair, lower your hips to knee level, and then straighten back up. You can feel your muscles working along with the internal and exterior rotators and the other butt and thigh muscle groups during all these actions.

Figure 7-10:
Your biggest
and most
powerful
muscles are
in your
lower body.

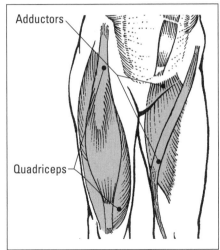
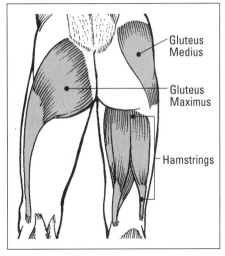

Part III
Cross-Training Plans

The 5th Wave   **By Rich Tennant**

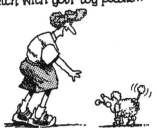

YOUR WEIGHTS ARE TOO LIGHT...

...if on any one routine you're doing more than 700 repetitions...

...if you can use them to play fetch with your toy poodle...

...if they keep getting lost in your wife's/husband's jewelry/cuff link drawer.

©RICHTENNANT

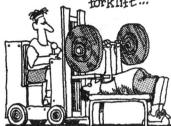

YOUR WEIGHTS ARE TOO HEAVY...

...if any part of your body explodes during a routine...

...if people refuse to spot for you without the aid of a forklift...

...if anywhere on your weights there appears the name of a ship and the word, "BALLAST".

In this part . . .

We lead you on the path to cross-training nirvana. This is it — the personalized workout system you've been waiting for! We've put together four different 12-week plans that will help you train for a number of different goals by giving you a comprehensive fitness prescription for all the elements of fitness that should be included in a cross-training program. Start by reading Chapter 8 to understand how the plans are structured. Then you can choose the plan you'd like to follow. If you're in doubt or are new to exercise, always start with the Base Fitness Plan. For a longer term approach, you can add plan after plan.

For each plan, we give you a specific weekly prescription to follow for 12 weeks. This includes a recommendation for the cardio, strength, and flexibility components of your plan, plus we pull out goal-specific exercises.

Chapter 8

How to Follow the Plans

. . . .

In This Chapter

▶ How to follow the plans

▶ How to modify the plans

▶ Five workout reminders

. . . .

*W*e know you're itching to get moving, but before you start, get smart: Choose the right plan to help you achieve your specific goal. In this chapter, we show you how to follow our workout prescription system. After you pick your plan, go over all the charts and notes to get a thorough understanding of what your workout schedule will be.

In Each Plan

Each plan — Base Fitness, Weight Loss, and Athletic — have some common elements. Each 12-week program, which varies every four weeks, contains

✔ A cardio stamina prescription that suggests what to do and how long and how often to do it.

✔ A muscle strength prescription with a recommended number of sets, repetitions, and days per week to perform the exercises.

✔ A flexibility prescription for the number of days a week to include the stretches from Chapters 15 or 28.

✔ A power prescription, if it's relevant to the plan, to include any explosive movements in your routine. ***Remember:*** Perform these high-intensity exercises only if you are injury-free, have developed a good base level of fitness, and have your doctor's okay.

✔ A skills prescription, if it's relevant to the plan, to help you develop speed, agility, and coordination.

✔ Rest prescriptions, which may include gentler activities that can keep you stimulated on your days off.

✔ Eight suggested muscle strength exercises, plus options for each, from Part IV.

✔ Recommendations on how to progress once you've completed the first 12-week cycle.

How to Follow the Plans

Ready to find out more? Follow these steps to learn about your program's basics:

1. **Choose a plan to follow, depending upon your goal.**

   If in doubt, always start with the Base Fitness Plan. It will help you develop all-around stamina and strength. You can then move on to another plan. Or you can repeat the same plan again, only this time varying it by changing the way you exercise and the exercises and activities that you do. Three shorter one-month cycles divide the 12-week cycle. Your exercise prescription will change slightly every four weeks to keep you challenged, but feel free to shorten your time following a certain prescription if you don't feel ready to move on. Likewise, you can push a little harder or lengthen your workouts if you feel capable of more.

2. **Each plan includes a chart that gives you an overview of what to do and when to do it. Use that chart to create a schedule that fits your lifestyle.**

   Your plan may suggest to do a cardio workout four times a week and a strength training workout three times a week. This doesn't mean that you should exercise seven days a week. Instead, couple up the items in the chart. On Day 1 of your weekly plan you might do the stretches, 20 minutes of cardio, and the 30-minute strength routine. On Day 3 of your plan, you might do only the strength exercises. Remember, rest days are an important — and necessary — part of your program.

   You have some flexibility, just keep within the training guidelines: Strength training should be done every other day, with a rest day in between to allow your muscles time to recover. Cardio activities should be varied, especially if you're including high-impact, high-intensity options like running. Power activities should be done only once a week and for a brief time. They should not be attempted unless you have developed a good base level of fitness and are injury-free. The skills drills can be done as often as every day, depending upon what they are. You won't need recovery time from a session spent doing simple ball drills or practicing free throws. However, you will need a day or two of rest after a series of wind sprints.

   Once you've figured out how to spread out your workouts, plan them into your schedule. You need to figure out what time and what days of the week are most convenient, and then slot in the appropriate activity.

It's always a good idea to schedule your weekly workouts in advance because even the most devout can easily slip into *Seinfeld*-rerun-mode and completely forget to hit the gym.

Remember that your rest days are considered workout days as well — or more precisely nonworkout days. They're integral to the plan because these are the days that your body responds to all that exercise stimulus by getting stronger. You can choose to do *active rest* days as well, where you simply do something for the fun of it, providing that it's easy on your body. Play Ping-Pong (and develop your hand-eye coordination) or stretch (flexible muscles are happy muscles).

3. Pick your activities.

We suggest some cardio activities in the notes for each plan. However, you can do whatever you like. All we ask is that you stick to the cross-training philosophy and choose at least two different cardio activities to do within your 12-week cycle. This is especially important if you're on a cardio intensive plan where you might be exercising five or six days a week. Overuse injuries are the result of doing the same old thing too often, so line up some options and keep it varied.

Which cardio activities you pick may have an effect on the planning you did in Step 2. If you've decided to ride your bike around the neighborhood, lifting weights at the gym might not be compatible, unless (hey!) you ride your bike to the gym. Revert back to Step 2 and make sure your plan is still convenient, based on the activities you've chosen.

We suggest eight key muscle strength exercises per plan. We designed these plan-specific moves to help you work toward your overall goal. You'll see pictures of the exercises and step-by-step instructions of how to do them in the chapters noted. Check to see that all of these moves are suitable for you. If they are too difficult to perform, or you have an injury or weakness that prevents you from performing a particular movement, try the option we've given or substitute your own move.

4. Find your range.

We give you a range to work within during your different activities. So if your cardio prescription says 15-25 minutes, aim to limit your workout to this amount of time. If you're a beginner, stay within the beginning of the range.

How long you work out also depends on your intensity. Overall, we recommend that you stay within a Target Heart Rate zone, working between 55 percent and 70 percent of your maximum. This corresponds to Levels 3-5 on the Perceived Rate of Exertion scale (see Chapter 6). If you're following the Athletic Plan or are exceptionally fit, you can work harder. If you do, you may want to shorten the workout time since exercising at a higher intensity will cause you to fatigue sooner. Think of alternating how you work out: either shorter sessions/harder intensity or lower intensity/longer sessions.

5. **Plug in the variables: You should modify the plan according to your own needs and limitations.**

   The fitness tests in Chapter 5 will help you pinpoint weaker and stronger areas that you might want to factor into your plan. If you're especially inflexible, you may want to add a few more stretching days. If your balance is poor, you might want to include as many standing exercises as you can to improve.

   The Mix-n-Match Plan is one that you create yourself based on the information throughout the book. You can make this highly specific, such as "I want to improve my tennis game," or general, such as "I want to feel fit." We give you general guidelines to follow to determine how often to do each type of exercise. If you're unsure of how to structure your plan, use the recommendations in the Base Fitness Plan, but plug in your individual choices for exercises and activities instead. When choosing a group of strength exercises, try to choose a well-balanced selection to target all your major muscle groups. We divide all the moves in the book according to upper body, lower body, and core abs and back to help you choose. Some of the multimuscle exercises will target several areas, however.

6. **Once you've finished your initial cross-training cycle, you can progress to the next level.**

   If you found the plan too progressive the first time around, you can follow the same plan again, but use shorter exercise periods and lighter weights this time around. Or you can simply repeat the same cycle again with other slight variations, such as switching activities and exercises that you do. You can also go to a completely new plan. Check out the Cheat Sheet at the front of the book or Chapter 3 for the many ways to cross-train. One easy way to up the ante is simply to switch the order of your strength exercises and perhaps add one new cardio activity to your routine. You don't have to get too technical to experience the body-changing benefits of cross-training.

   Look at your training as a series of different levels that you must achieve before moving on. First, you want to make sure that you've built up good levels of general strength, stamina, and flexibility. If you have these, the next level — where you push yourself by working harder, faster, and/or more often — will come easier. Once you've upped the ante, you can shift your focus from fitness to performance, working on more functional movements and skills that will help you excel at specific activities. You may want to incorporate maintenance periods as well, where you give your body a break from more challenges and try to maintain the level you've achieved. See Chapter 3 for more information on switching up your routine.

Choosing a Plan

This section can help you select a plan that fits your goals. Remember that each plan can be custom-made to suit you depending upon which activities and exercises you choose to do. We provide a general prescription so that you can get an idea of the frequency and types of exercises to do.

Base Fitness Plan

This plan is good for those who want a solid starting point and those who have not exercised regularly in two months or longer. But remember, any plan can be modified to decrease or increase the difficulty to better suit you. All you need to do is decrease the time and intensity of each activity, switch to easier exercises, or perform easier modifications of them.

The Base Fitness Plan focuses on developing a standard level of fitness. Depending upon which end of the range of exercise time and repetitions you choose, the routine can lean toward harder, more intense workouts, or easier, lighter workouts. This is the plan you should follow if you're a beginner or an experienced exerciser, wanting to get back onto a scheduled routine and making sure you develop good all-round fitness before pushing yourself to higher levels of activity. See Chapter 9 for the Base Fitness Plan.

Weight Loss Plan

The Weight Loss Plan is a more time-intensive plan geared toward burning more calories through more cardio work and increasing the metabolism over the long term through an intense circuit routine of strength moves. The Weight Loss Plan is great for those who are fit enough to exercise more frequently and at a slightly higher intensity. The added time and exercise days will help decrease body fat and improve body shape. See Chapter 10 for the Weight Loss Plan.

Athletic Plan

If you'd like to improve your performance in a particular sport or fitness activity such as running, cycling, or skiing, this is the plan for you. This plan is also helpful for those who have become fit through standard gym and cardio work and would like to develop athletic skills.

The Athletic Plan switches the focus to the power and skill side of the fitness equation. You'll do a minimal level of cardio and strength work, but most of your effort will be geared toward becoming faster, more agile, more powerful, and more adept at those skills specific to your sport, whether it's slaloms in skiing, serves in tennis, or throwing in softball. Because this plan involves some explosive power exercises (see Chapter 20), don't push yourself to these levels unless you're already in very good shape, have a good level of strength, and have no existing joint injuries or weakness. If, during the fitness tests in Chapter 5, you found that you were weak in the stability, balance, and back tests, strengthen these areas first with a solid program of weight exercises before attempting these high-stress moves. See Chapter 11 for the Athletic Plan.

Mix-n-Match Plan

If you're comfortable with the concept of cross-training, are familiar with basic fitness schedules, and want to design a plan to best suit your needs, you might want to follow the Mix-n-Match Plan.

The Mix-n-Match Plan can comprise as many cardio activities as you like, although we recommend choosing at least two to four during the course of each 12-week cycle. You can tailor your strength routine according to the moves you enjoy doing most. We separate the moves down into different areas of the body that are worked. Pick two to three moves from each group to target all your major muscle groups. See Chapter 12 for more information about the Mix-n-Match Plan and step-by-step instructions on creating your own plan.

Modifying the Plans

The plans we provide are simply a palate upon which you can add your signature touch. If you find your enthusiasm waning and your body getting used to the same moves, you'll need to make slight modifications to your daily sessions as well as your weekly and monthly schedules.

You can make sweeping changes — try a whole new cardio activity, for example — or you can make minor adjustments to the way you work out — do two more reps per set, add a pound or two to your weight, add 5 more minutes of cardio, or subtract 10 minutes but up the intensity. Break up a 45-minute session into three 15-minute bouts. Work with rubber tubing instead of weights.

Below are some suggestions, but you can also check out Chapter 3 for more ideas. Keep this book next to your cross-trainers, so when you're ready to lace them up, you can flip through and find a quick tip to add a little pizzazz to your workout each day:

✔ Mix different activities together during the same session.

✔ Create a mini-circuit, alternating strength and cardio moves.

✔ Use different fitness equipment: stability balls, exercise bands, balance boards, a step, medicine balls, dumbbells, barbells, weighted bars, weighted vests, or fitness tubing.

✔ Switch cardio intensities: Alternate shorter, harder workouts with longer, slower workouts. Or try *Fartlek sprints,* a training method named after the Swedish word for "speed play." You alternate bursts of exercise with slower, recovery intervals by speeding up and slowing down intermittently during your cardio workout.

✔ Substitute a new sport for one of your cardio sessions.

✔ Intensify your weight routine: increase the weight and decrease the number of reps, or decrease the weight and add a few more reps.

✔ Superset your moves: Change the order of moves you do within a set and group them together in pairs of two or three and perform them with little rest in between.

Workout reminders

Even a pro can get sloppy when it comes to exercise. Here are our key tips that you should keep in mind:

✔ **Listen to your body:** If something hurts, stop the exercise. Or if you're not getting much of a workout, give yourself a little push.

✔ **Be patient:** Don't try to do too much too soon. If you take it slow, you'll be much more likely to stick to the program and experience longer-lasting, healthier physical changes.

✔ **Be prepared:** Wear the right shoes and clothing, and use the right protective equipment for each activity.

✔ **Concentrate on form:** It's easy to let power overtake technique. You may be strong enough to lift a heavier weight with poor form than a lighter weight with perfect form. But it's more important to develop control and precision before pushing yourself to physical extremes. Over the long run, if you slow things down and focus on the quality of your movement, whether it's a basketball serve, an aerobics move, or a weights exercise, you'll have fewer injuries and will have more power from doing it correctly. See Chapter 13 for information on technique.

✔ **Keep it varied:** Since variety is the buzzword in cross-training, we can't remind you enough. Keep it interesting for your body and your mind. See Chapter 3 for some tips and tricks of the trade.

Chapter 9

Base Fitness Plan

*1*f you're ready to lace up your shoes and flex your muscles, this is the chapter for you! First read Chapter 8 to find out how the plans work. This Base Fitness Plan focuses on developing a standard level of fitness. This is the plan you should follow if you're a beginner or if you're an experienced exerciser wanting to get back onto a scheduled routine. (Make sure you develop a good all-round fitness before pushing yourself to higher levels of activity.)

Let's Get Started

We divide this 12-week program into three shorter 1-month cycles. Your exercise prescription will change slightly every four weeks to keep you challenged, but feel free to lengthen your time following a certain prescription if you're feeling ready to move on. If you're not feeling up to the challenge, give yourself a break every once in a while, especially in the beginning. Pushing yourself too hard when you're not feeling well will only result in an increased risk for injuries or burnout. And who can get in shape when you're plagued with painful problems or ready to quit?

Table 9-1 outlines the Base Fitness Plan. See the sections following the table for suggestions on how to incorporate exercises into the plan.

Table 9-1	The Base Cross-Training Plan on a 12-Week Cycle		
	Month 1	*Month 2*	*Month 3*
CARDIO STAMINA	3 sessions a week for 15-25 minutes per session	4 sessions a week for 25-40 minutes per session	5 sessions a week for 45-60 minutes per session
MUSCLE STRENGTH	2-3 sessions a week. Do 2 sets of 8-12 repetitions of each selected exercise	3 sessions a week. Do 3 sets of 8-12 repetitions of each selected exercise	3 sessions a week. Do 3 sets of 8-12 repetitions of each selected exercise
FLEXIBILITY	3 sessions a week; pick 6-10 exercises	3 sessions a week; pick 6-10 exercises	3 sessions a week; pick 6-10 exercises
POWER	No power moves should be done in the first month	No power moves should be done in the second month	1 short session a week
SKILLS	No skills drills should be done in the first month	No skills drills should be done in the second month	1 session a week

Cardio

You can choose from a variety of activities to fulfill your cardio requirement. You can run, walk, take fitness classes, or play a sport like soccer, for example. Check out Part V for ideas. Aim to mix up the types of activities you do so that you don't always do the exact same workout, and shoot for an intensity where you feel like you're working somewhat hard or at Level 3-4 on the Perceived Rate of Exertion scale (see Chapter 6).

Muscle strength exercises

To build your muscle strength, try these exercises following the suggested schedule in Table 9-1. Start with dumbbells that are 5-10 pounds, and progress to heavier weight when the last few repetitions of each set become easy. (Review Chapters 7 and 14 to update yourself on weight lifting technique.) Do the whole set of exercises at once. Remember you can substitute any exercises that you do not feel comfortable doing.

Exercises	*Options*
Squat (see Chapter 16)	Plié squat (see Chapter 16)
Push-up (see Chapter 16)	Triceps dip (see Chapter 16)
Walk-thru lunge (see Chapter 18)	Back lunge (see Chapter 16)
Rubber band row (see Chapter 17)	Lat pull
Side lunge (see Chapter 18)	Standing side leg lift (see Chapter 17)
Biceps curl (see Chapter 17)	Squat curl (see Chapter 18)
Bentover deltoid (see Chapter 17)	Lateral raise (see Chapter 17)
Ab curl (see Chapter 16)	Reverse curl (see Chapter 16)

Flexibility

To improve your flexibility, follow the suggested times in Table 9-1, and run through the moves in Chapter 15. Pick 6-10 exercises that target all your major muscle groups. You can also run through the bench stretches in Chapter 28.

Power

Once you have finished the first two cycles (months 1 and 2), you may be ready to begin working on your power. ***Remember:*** You should have yourself re-evaluated by a doctor or fitness professional before starting these new moves, as some are very advanced moves and you may need more time to work up to them. See Chapter 20 for descriptions of the moves you're going to use. You should try the jump lunge and slalom twist for starters. Power workouts should be short and sweet. For the number of repetitions that you should do, see suggestions in the directions for each move in Chapter 20.

Sports skills

After completing the first two months, you should be ready to try some of the sports drills outlined in Chapter 21. These drills test your speed, agility, and coordination, making you a stronger and faster athlete. *Remember:* It's a good idea to get re-evaluated for your level of fitness before trying these moves. Try the straight line cone drill, the zigzag drill, and the dancer's leap for starters.

Active rest

Consider your rest days as workout days as well. Alternate between taking total rest days — where you truly minimize your physical activity, especially if you've had an intense week of workouts — and active rest days, where you can do some sort of gentle, light activity. You can choose to simply do something for the fun of it, providing that it's easy on your body. Play badminton or Ping-Pong, bowl, stretch, or go for an easy bike ride. *Remember:* Your rest days are integral to the plan because your body responds to all that exercise stimulus by getting stronger on these days.

After Three Months . . .

Increase the intensity of your cardio workouts. Check out Chapter 6 for ways to do this. You can move faster, push yourself harder to work at a higher intensity, or substitute a higher intensity activity (running for walking, for example).

To keep getting stronger first increase the amount of weight you use, dropping back to completing just 1-2 sets if you need to, and then increase the number of sets you do. Also try new exercises. Read Chapter 14 for details on weight lifting technique.

Chapter 10

Weight Loss Plan

· ·

In This Chapter

▶ Getting started on the plan

▶ Moving forward after three months

· ·

*I*f your goal is to fight the flab, this 12-week program is for you. The Weight Loss Plan focuses on burning lots of calories in the short term through intensive and frequent cardio work. It focuses on boosting your metabolism in the long term through a comprehensive total-body weight lifting program.

Let's Get Started

For the muscle strength exercises we recommend as part of the plan, we pair up exercises and insert high-intensity cardio intervals to create a strength circuit routine. This maximizes the fat-burning effectiveness of your moves. Studies show that strength circuit intervals are one of the best ways to burn calories. Think of it as the exercise diet where you burn up more than you can eat.

Don't be fooled: This is not a walk in the park. For exercise to have significant body changing effects, it must be frequent and intensive — so you should be fit and healthy enough to withstand longer sessions or cope with a high frequency of workouts where you will be exercising intensely for up to five days a week. If you're a beginner, you can still follow this plan, but you may want to work in the lower ranges of the exercise prescriptions. Draw out the plans by spending two months on each month-long cycle; shorten the sessions and expect changes to come a little slower. Or you can start with the Base Fitness Plan and move onto this plan afterward.

Table 10-1 outlines the Weight Loss Plan. See the sections following the table for suggestions on how to add exercises into the plan.

Table 10-1	Weight Loss Plan on a 12-Week Cycle		
	Month 1	*Month 2*	*Month 3*
CARDIO STAMINA	3-5 sessions a week for 20-30 minutes per session	5 sessions a week for 35-45 minutes per session	5-6 sessions a week for 45-60 minutes per session
MUSCLE STRENGTH	3 sessions a week. Do 2 sets of 8 repetitions of each selected exercise	3 sessions a week. Do 2 sets of 10 repetitions of each selected exercise	3 sessions a week. Do 3 sets of 10 repetitions of each selected exercise
FLEXIBILITY	3 sessions a week; pick 6-10 exercises	3 sessions a week; pick 6-10 exercises	3 sessions a week; pick 6-10 exercises
POWER	No power moves should be done in the first month	No power moves should be done in the second month	1 short session a week
SKILLS	No skills drills should be done in the first month	No skills drills should be done in the second month	1 session a week

Cardio

Aim for an intensity where you feel like you are working somewhat hard to hard or at Level 4-6 on the Perceived Rate of Exertion scale (see Chapter 6). During the cardio portions of the circuit workout, your intensity should be hard to very hard for maximum calorie-burning benefits. As always, slow down if you're feeling fatigued. Stop if you're feeling lightheaded or dizzy.

Choose high-intensity cardio options such as running, inline skating, aerobics, or cardio machines. Check out Part V for ideas on all the activities you can include.

Muscle strength exercises

To build your muscle strength, start with dumbbells that are 5-15 pounds. These moves should be done in order as a quick circuit. You can work up to heavier weights if you do not feel like the muscles are being sufficiently fatigued (see Chapters 7 and 14). Complete one set of the first three moves in order, trying not to rest in between. Then do a two-minute cardio interval of jumping jacks, jumping rope, jogging in place, or stepping on and off a low step before going on to the next superset of three combined exercises. Insert another two-minute cardio interval and complete the third superset, followed by a final two-minute interval. Then run through the entire group one more time. Try to rest no longer than 60 seconds in between supersets.

We include a significant amount of multimuscle, combo upper and lower body moves in this routine. If this is too difficult, choose the easier options listed.

Exercises	*Options*
Squat curl (see Chapter 18)	Biceps curl (see Chapter 17)
Push-up (see Chapter 16)	Triceps dip (see Chapter 17)
Weighted walking lunge (see Chapter 18)	Plié squat (see Chapter 16)
2 minutes of jumping jacks	2 minutes of marching in place
Reverse curl (see Chapter 16)	Ab twist on ball (see Chapter 17)
Standing side leg lift (see Chapter 17)	Single leg extension (see Chapter 17)
Squat press (see Chapter 18)	Military press overhead (see Chapter 17)
2 minutes jumping rope	2 minutes of standing knee lifts
Lunge scissor kick (see Chapter 18)	Walk-thru lunge (see Chapter 18)
Chop squat (see Chapter 18)	Slalom jump twist (see Chapter 20)
2 minutes of step-ups	2 minutes of stepping side to side

Flexibility

To get more flexible, follow the suggested times in Table 10-1, and run through the moves in Chapter 15. Pick 6-10 exercises that target your major muscles groups, or run through the bench stretches in Chapter 28.

Power

Once you have finished the first two cycles (months 1 and 2), you may be ready to begin working on your power. We include a couple of options for you in the preceding list of recommended muscle strength exercises. ***Remember:*** You should have yourself re-evaluated by a doctor or fitness professional before starting these new moves, as some are very advanced moves and you may need more time to work up to them. See Chapter 20 for descriptions of the moves you're going to use.

Sports skills

After completing the first two months, you should be ready to try some of the sports drills outlined in Chapter 21. These drills test your speed, agility, and coordination. Because many involve sprinting, they will burn a lot of calories fast. However, they are more difficult too, so make sure that you are fit enough to push yourself to work at a higher intensity. ***Remember:*** It's a good idea to get re-evaluated for your level of fitness before trying these moves. Try the zigzag drill and the square cone drill for starters.

Active rest

Consider your rest days as workout days as well. Alternate between taking total rest days — where you truly minimize your physical activity, especially if you've had an intense week of workouts — and active rest days where you can do some sort of gentle, light activity. You can choose to simply do something for the fun of it, providing that it's easy on your body. Go for a low intensity, long walk or leisurely, but lengthy, bike ride. ***Remember:*** Your rest days are integral to the plan because your body responds to all that exercise stimulus by getting stronger on these days.

After Three Months . . .

Increase the intensity and duration of your cardio workouts. Check out Chapter 6 for ways to do this. You can move faster, push yourself harder to work at a higher intensity, or substitute a higher intensity activity (running for walking, for example). When you increase the length of your cardio session, you might want to go a little easier and work at a lower intensity.

In your circuit routine, increase the amount of weight you use, dropping to 1-2 sets if you need to, and then increase the number of sets you do to three. Read Chapter 14 for details on weight lifting technique.

Chapter 11

Athletic Plan

*Y*ou can be fit enough to run a marathon, but that doesn't do you much good if your real goal is to hit a home run, have agility on the tennis court, or improve your swimming technique in a triathlon. Make no mistake, when it comes to sports, training must be highly specific. A fit, strong, flexible body will help you perform well; however, you must exceed this basic level of fitness and hone those skills and abilities that are required for your chosen activity in order to excel.

One thing to keep in mind is that, while gym fitness is designed to take out all the risky variables like slippery floors and people that bump into you, this is not the case with sports and competitive activities. Whether it's football, ballet, or running, the intense nature of the discipline — when approached in a semi-professional or competitive way — means that there are risks. Many sports contain explosive movements, sudden changes of direction, bodies slamming against hard objects or other bodies, and excessive force on certain joints due to actions like throwing and kicking. It stands to reason that the stronger your body is, the more capable your body is of withstanding these unpredictable or excessive forces safely. It also means that you might have to do some training that is more intense than the average person. Plyometric movements are one example of a sports-specific training technique that is difficult and can be risky, but when incorporated carefully into a safe, well-rounded training program, can also enhance your sports performance.

Let's Get Started

You should have already developed a good base level of fitness to follow this plan. If you're out-of-shape and found more than two weaknesses while taking the fitness tests in Chapter 5, you should follow the Base Fitness Plan first and improve your fitness level before tackling this high-intensity plan.

This plan follows a standard formula we created. Since every sport is unique, you'll have to determine which sport-specific moves and drills to do in order to get the best results for your chosen activity. If in doubt, follow the plan as it is outlined and make modifications once you're familiar with the cross-training system.

Note: One major point of difference compared to the other plans is that the Athletic Plan switches the focus to the power and skill side of your fitness routine. You'll do a minimal level of cardio and strength work, because most of your effort will be geared toward becoming faster, more agile, and more powerful. Don't push yourself to these levels unless you are already in very good shape, have a good level of strength, and have no existing joint injuries or weakness.

Table 11-1 outlines the Athletic Plan. See the sections following the table for suggestions on how to incorporate exercises into the plan.

Table 11-1	The Athletic Plan on a 12-Week Cycle		
	Month 1	**Month 2**	**Month 3**
CARDIO STAMINA	3 sessions a week for 15-25 minutes per session	3 sessions a week for 15-25 minutes per session	3 sessions a week for 15-25 minutes per session
MUSCLE STRENGTH	3 sessions a week. Do 2 sets of 8-12 repetitions of each selected exercise.	3 sessions a week. Do 3 sets of 8-12 repetitions of each selected exercise.	3 sessions a week. Do 3 sets of 8-12 repetitions of each selected exercise.
FLEXIBILITY	3 sessions a week; pick 6-10 exercises	3 sessions a week; pick 6-10 exercises	3 sessions a week; pick 6-10 exercises
POWER	1 short session a week.	1 short session a week.	1 short session a week.
SKILLS	4 sessions a week.	4 sessions a week.	4 sessions a week.

Cardio

Aim for an intensity where you feel like you are working hard to very hard or at Level 5-7 on the Perceived Rate of Exertion scale (see Chapter 6). Choose the cardio activities that best complement your sport (see Part V if in doubt).

Muscle strength exercises

To build muscle strength, start with dumbbells that are 10-15 pounds. See Part V for sport-specific moves, or choose the following. Make sure that you are injury-free before performing any plyometric exercises.

Exercises	Options
Squat (see Chapter 16)	Back lunge (see Chapter 16)
Push-up (see Chapter 16)	Chest press (see Chapter 19)
Military press overhead (see Chapter 17)	Plié squat with raise (see Chapter 18)
Lat pulldown (see Chapter 19)	Rubber band row (see Chapter 17)
Ab crunch on ball (see Chapter 17)	Reverse curl (see Chapter 16)
Single leg extension (see Chapter 17)	Back extension (see Chapter 17)
Jump lunge (see Chapter 20)	Lunge scissor kick (see Chapter 18)
Burst jump (see Chapter 20)	Depth jump (see Chapter 20)

Flexibility

Run through the moves in Chapter 15 to improve your flexibility. Pick out 6-10 exercises to target your major muscle groups, or run through the bench stretches in Chapter 28. Also, make sure to check out Part V. We suggest specific stretches that will help you target muscle groups that are used during specific sports.

Power

We include exercises for you to try in the recommended muscle strength exercises above. *Remember:* You should have yourself re-evaluated by a doctor or fitness professional before starting these new moves, as some are very advanced moves and you may need more time to work up to them. See Chapter 20 for descriptions of the moves you're going to use and for the number of repetitions that you should do.

Sports skills

Choose the agility drills that best complement your sport in Part V and find out how to do them in Chapter 21. These drills test your speed, agility, and coordination. Make sure that you are fit enough to push yourself to work at a higher intensity. *Remember:* It's a good idea to get re-evaluated for your level of fitness before trying these moves.

Active rest

You work hard, but ya gotta rest easy. Alternate between taking total rest days, where you truly minimize your physical activity, and active rest days, where you can do some sort of gentle, light activity. You can choose to simply do something for the fun of it, providing that it's easy on your body. Stretch, or go for an easy swim or bike ride on your days off. *Remember:* Your rest days are integral to the plan because your body responds to all that exercise stimulus by getting stronger on these days.

After Three Months . . .

Get specific training advice from a coach for your sport to further enhance your skills. To find a coach, check out the organizations for your favorite sport in Appendix B.

Chapter 12

Mix-n-Match Plan

· ·

In This Chapter

▶ Getting started

▶ Choosing activities

▶ Following research guidelines

▶ Organizing your schedule

▶ Thinking of the long term

· ·

*A*re you ready to become the master of your own destiny? Well, pick up a
pencil, put on your cross-trainers, and get ready to shake that body into
shape! You can design your own cross-training plan using the guidelines we
give in this chapter. (If you're new to exercise, or haven't been on a regular
schedule for a long time, we recommend that you follow the Base Fitness
Plan in Chapter 9 first.) With the Mix-n-Match plan, you can simply plug in the
activities that suit your goal well. We designed this plan to help you work
toward a highly specific aim — you'd like to become more coordinated or
develop special skills, for example — or if you have specific limitations — all
of your cardio work must be low impact, or if you have limited access to a
gym. This plan can help you individualize your routine so that it suits you. It
takes a little brainwork because you'll have to decide which activities will
best develop the skills you want to improve, and you'll have to designate the
appropriate times, intensity, and other training variables. Our step-by-step
guidelines will help you determine how to structure your schedule.

The Mix-n-Match plan can include as many cardio activities as you like,
although we recommend choosing two to four during the course of each 12-
week cycle. You can tailor your strength routine according to the moves you
enjoy doing most. Go through the moves in Part IV to become familiar with
the technique and the muscle groups that are targeted. Review the activities
in Part V, taking careful note of moves we identify as being especially good for
a particular sport or activity that you wish to do. We separate the exercises
into the different areas of the body that are worked. Pick three to four moves
from each group to target all your major muscle groups. (Review the muscle
groups in Chapter 7.)

Creating Your Plan Step by Step

Here's an overview of your step-by-step plan:

1. **Make long-term and short-term goals.**

2. **Set a time frame.**

3. **(Optional) Take the fitness tests to measure your progress later.**

4. **List activities that you feel comfortable doing and enjoy. Now, list new activities you'd like to try. Out of these two lists, choose activities to implement into your plan.**

5. **Plan your schedule using research guidelines from the American College of Sports Medicine and other institutions (see the chart later in this chapter).**

6. **Choose your exercises for each fitness section — cardio stamina, muscle strength, power, flexibility, and sports skills.**

7. **Figure in your active rest days.**

8. **Plan for the future by following steps to create a long-term plan.**

Each one of these steps is broken down into individual sections.

Making Goals

When pinpointing what it is exactly that you're trying to accomplish, be aware of how big and practical your goal is. If you want to improve the way you look, is it inches you want to lose or do you just need to firm up? If you want to feel more energetic, is it so that you have more energy in your daily life or so that you feel very powerful when you perform an endurance activity? Are you less interested in the body changing properties of exercise and more interested in how it's a great way to release the tension of your day? Or are you simply bored with your current routine and want to make a change? How much and what type of exercise you do will depend on your aims. Write down your main long-term goal. Then make smaller short-term goals in order of importance. Then pick your most important short-term goal and make it S.M.A.R.T. (specific, measurable, attainable, realistic, and timed). (See Chapter 4 for more about setting goals.)

Long-term goal: _____

Short-term goal 1: _____

Short-term goal 2: _____

Short-term goal 3: _____

Setting a Time Frame

Are you trying to get in shape for summer, look better in time for your ten-year high school reunion, or train for a triathlon that's four months away? Keeping in mind how much time you're able to dedicate to your workouts each week, how consistent you are sticking to them, and what shape you are in to begin with, will all affect how long it takes you to reach your goal. Small, simple goals are easier to achieve. Big goals often require more challenging and more frequent workouts (and you need to be fit enough to handle them).

How much time a day/week/month can you spend or are you willing to spend working out? Be realistic. Place your answer on line A. If you know that you simply are unable to commit to a schedule of say, four times a week, be aware that you may have to adjust your expectations: It may take you longer to reach your goal, depending upon what it is. It might be that you can sneak in little bits of exercise elsewhere to compensate for the day or two that you'll miss. If your goal is to improve your health, minimal levels of regular activity will help, but if you're trying to improve in some way athletically, your results may be compromised by not being able to dedicate the proper amount of time to training. When are the ideal times that you would like to exercise? Insert your answer on line B. When are the times that you know you can commit to a schedule without being interrupted? Insert your answer on line C.

A. _____

B. _____

C. _____

Taking the Fitness Tests

Using the home fitness tests from Chapter 5, pinpoint what area of fitness you may need to work on: cardio, flexibility, endurance, strength, and so on. Based on what you learned in Chapters 2, 6, and 7, determine what type of exercise you need to do to improve this area. Develop your entire plan from your weakest point outward. You're only as strong as your weakest link. So, for example, if you have poor upper body strength but tremendous muscular endurance in your legs, choose some exercises to go along with your running and cycling program that will benefit your upper body. We suggest adding some strength training exercises. You can also add rowing and swimming to balance out the lower body emphasis of your cardio workouts.

Even if you don't find any specific area to work on, using the fitness tests as a marker to measure your progress after you've completed the first 12-week phase of your plan is a good way to inspire yourself to go for the next 12-week plan!

Choosing Activities

You could probably try a new fitness activity every week of the year, but although part of the cross-training philosophy is that you try new things, it's important to keep those activities that you already enjoy in your plan. If it's not broken, don't fix it. List the exercises that you enjoy doing:

_____

_____

Now think of new activities you would like to try. The elliptical trainer? Tennis lessons? Mountain biking? Dance, boxing, judo, sports, or the many types of fitness classes? Flip through Part V to see if anything strikes your fancy. Add those new activities here:

_____

_____

From your list of new and current activities, consider your goals and choose two to four activities that you want to include in your schedule during the first 12 weeks. Start with base activities that you're most familiar with, and then add one new one as you feel ready. Don't give yourself too much to learn at one time. You don't have to overload yourself.

Organizing Your Schedule

Now you need to organize your sessions. The American College of Sports Medicine and other academic and research institutions conduct and review research done in different areas of fitness. Based on the cumulative findings, you should follow their general recommendations on how much and how often to do different types of exercise. Review each set of the following recommendations, and plan your schedule to stay within the suggested exercise prescriptions. You have some flexibility when it comes to exercise. It's more important that you do something — anything — and stick to it, than follow a very strict, rigid program for three weeks and then drop out for five.

If you have a week where you don't make all your sessions, just follow the same routine next week, adding a little more intensity or a few extra minutes onto your workouts if you can to make up some of what you missed. In general, the less you do, the smaller your results. If you're extremely fit and you're seeking high levels of fitness, you may need to push yourself to the upper ranges of the guidelines.

First, read through the list to determine how often and how long you should be working out each exercise element, and then enter your numbers into Table 14-1:

✔ Do 20-60 minutes of continuous or intermittent cardio activities, 3-5 days a week. Exercising fewer than two days a week at too low of an intensity is not enough of a stimulus to elicit a training effect. Moderate intensity exercise performed for an accumulated 30 minutes almost every day will provide significant health benefits, but may not help you reach the more competitive fitness levels.

Training intensity should be with 55 to 90 percent of maximum heart rate, or Level 3-8 on the Perceived Rate of Exertion scale (see Chapter 6). Working out at the highest intensities is only recommended for healthy adults training for athletic competition. Working out at the lowest intensities is recommended for those who are quite unfit. Keep the faith here, if you are out of shape and want to get into killer aerobic condition, start at the lower end of the intensity range and gradually progress over the weeks and months to the higher end of the scale. Always keep your exercise relatively comfortable, be consistent with your habit, and above all listen to your body.

✔ Do at least one set of 8-12 repetitions of a range of exercises that target all the major muscle groups. The intensity, the amount of weight used, should be enough to make it somewhat difficult (but not impossible) to finish that last rep. This type of workout will enhance strength, build muscle, and increase muscular endurance. You should work out no more than two or three days a week with a rest day in between. If muscle groups are broken up and alternated, it is possible to train every day (for example, Mondays do arms and abs, Tuesdays do legs and back, and so on).

✔ Do at least two to three days a week to stretch the major muscle groups. Or you may find it easier simply to stretch for 5-10 minutes after warming up and after each workout session. Each stretch should be held for 10-60 seconds.

✔ Explosive jumps shouldn't be performed by those who are out of shape, have orthopedic limitations, or aren't training specifically for a sport or competitive activity that requires explosive strength. Limit power or plyometric training to one day a week and keep the repetitions to between 1-6 and the duration to less than one minute.

✔ Some skill drills are more difficult than others and more taxing to different areas of the body. To develop skills, repetition with the proper technique is crucial. However, overuse of a certain area of the body (throwing a pitch with the same arm, practicing a golf swing, or leaping off the same foot) can lead to injuries. Some techniques that are extremely demanding, such as cone drills that involve sprinting, may be considered a part of your cardio stamina or muscular strength workout, so follow the appropriate preceding guidelines.

Now, to fill in your chart, do the following: For cardio, determine the number of times you'll do cardio work during the week. Enter that number and the total time. For muscle strength, determine the number of times you'll do muscle strength exercises and enter the number of sets and reps into the table. For flexibility, power, and skills, just note how many times you'll work those elements during the week. Enter all these values in Table 14-1.

Table 14-1	**Your 12-Week Cycle**		
	Month 1	*Month 2*	*Month 3*
CARDIO STAMINA	__ sessions a week for __ minutes per session.	__ sessions a week for __ minutes per session.	__ sessions a week for __ minutes per session.
MUSCLE STRENGTH	__ sessions a week. Do __ sets of __ repetitions of each selected exercise.	__ sessions a week. Do __ sets of __ repetitions of each selected exercise.	__ sessions a week. Do __ sets of __ repetitions of each selected exercise.
FLEXIBILITY	__ sessions a week; pick 6-10 exercises and hold each one for 10-60 seconds.	__ sessions a week; pick 6-10 exercises and hold each one for 10-60 seconds.	__ sessions a week; pick 6-10 exercises and hold each one for 10-60 seconds.
POWER	__ sessions a week; keep repetitions to 1-6 and the duration to less than a minute.	__ sessions a week; keep repetitions to 1-6 and the duration to less than a minute.	__ sessions a week; keep repetitions to 1-6 and the duration to less than a minute.
SKILLS	__ sessions a week.	__ sessions a week.	__ sessions a week.

Choosing Specific Exercises from Each Fitness Section

Pick three or four exercises from each section — cardio stamina, muscle strength, power, flexibility, and skills — paying special attention to which muscle groups are worked, for a whole body workout. Review the activities in Part V, taking careful note of moves or drills that are especially good for a particular sport or activity that you wish to do.

Here are the exercises that'll work the lower body (buttocks and legs):

Exercise	Chapter You'll Find It In
Squat	Chapter 16
Plié squat	Chapter 16
Back lunge	Chapter 16
Single leg extension	Chapter 17
Standing side leg lift	Chapter 17
Walk-thru lunge	Chapter 18
Weighted walking lunge	Chapter 18
Side lunge	Chapter 18
Dynamic side lunge	Chapter 18
Squat press	Chapter 18
Squat curl	Chapter 18
Lunge scissor kick	Chapter 18
Chop squat	Chapter 18
One leg squat press	Chapter 18
Standing good morning	Chapter 18
Jump lunge	Chapter 20
Lateral hop	Chapter 20 (Do these only for advanced levels of sports-specific training.)
Slalom jump twist	Chapter 20

(continued)

Exercise	*Chapter You'll Find It In*
Depth jump	Chapter 20 (Do these only for advanced levels of sports-specific training.)
Burst jump	Chapter 20 (Do these only for advanced levels of sports-specific training.)

Choose from these exercises that work on your core (back and abs):

Exercise	*Chapter You'll Find It In*
Ab curl	Chapter 16
Reverse curl	Chapter 16
Push-up	Chapter 16
Bentover deltoid	Chapter 17
Military press overhead	Chapter 17
Ab crunch on ball	Chapter 17
Ab twist on ball	Chapter 17
Back extension	Chapter 17
Rubber band row	Chapter 17
Chop squat	Chapter 18
Standing good morning	Chapter 18
Lower body ball twist	Chapter 18
Reverse back extension	Chapter 19
Lat pulldown	Chapter 19

To work your upper body (arms, chest, and shoulders), choose exercises from this list:

Exercise	*Chapter You'll Find It In*
Plié squat	Chapter 16
Push-up	Chapter 16
Triceps dip	Chapter 16
Lateral raise	Chapter 17
Bentover deltoid	Chapter 17

Exercise	Chapter You'll Find It In
Military press overhead	Chapter 17
Triceps kickback	Chapter 17
Biceps curl	Chapter 17
Rubber band row	Chapter 17
Squat press	Chapter 18
Squat curl	Chapter 18
Incline chest press	Chapter 19
Triceps cable extension	Chapter 19
Lat pulldown	Chapter 19

Adding in Your Rest Days

Write down a few easy activities that you can do, from shopping to playing Ping-Pong, on your days off. This way, when you need to take a break, you'll still be keeping active. Remember, though, if you need a day off, take it! We want you to enjoy this, not make it a chore.

Thinking Long Term

When developing your own program, always remember the big picture because it will determine where you want to focus at different points in your plan. At various times you'll need to shift your focus on the various aspects of performance and fitness. Follow these basic steps to help you develop your fitness future:

1. **You want to make sure that you've developed a good base level of fitness.**

   This is true no matter how fit you are, because your base level will change according to your goal. For someone who wants to train for a marathon, for example, he'll have to establish a base fitness level of being able to run 20 or so miles a week before he can start pushing up the intensity and the mileage. Someone who wants to start running for fitness (not competition) will have to establish a base level of fitness that ensures that he can walk fast for at least 20 minutes before he can progress.

Don't underestimate our Base Fitness Plan in Chapter 9. You can manipulate where you fall on the fitness prescription scale to make it fit your beginning or advanced fitness level.

2. **You want to go through a growth cycle where you push yourself a little bit more.**

   This might mean increasing the number of reps and sets you do when lifting weights or it might mean lifting more weights. It could also mean increasing the speed at which you cycle or adding hills to your usual cycling path.

   You want to get a bit more specific if you have a particular sport or activity in mind that you're training for. You may want to ease off a little bit on the base fitness training and concentrate more on the performance skills: perfecting your catching and fielding ability, practicing free throws, improving your agility, becoming more powerful, and so on.

3. **Let your body have a maintenance period.**

   It's a good idea to have maintenance periods where you hold the intensity and duration of your activity constant. This allows your body to settle in on its new level of fitness. The amount of time you spend in maintenance is very individual and depends on your goals, motivation, and intuition. These periods can last from as little as a week to a few months. When you feel ready, turn up the intensity a bit, make some changes, or introduce new activities.

4. **Mix up the plan when you're due for a change. We recommend changing every 12-16 weeks.**

   Review your current plan and figure out what you can fiddle with to modify the stimulus. You can switch to a new cardio activity and substitute a new set of exercises and follow the same prescription. Or you can continue with the same moves and activities, but vary the intensity, weight, or number of sets or minutes you do.

Check out Chapter 3 for an introduction to periodization. It's the athlete's secret weapon to keeping injuries at bay and keeping things interesting.

Remember: You should have a base level of fitness already. Please see your doctor before embarking on the next fitness level.

Part IV
Fabulous Moves

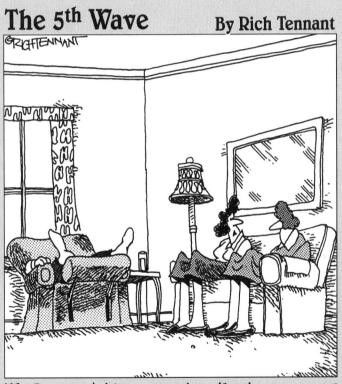

The 5th Wave   By Rich Tennant

"No, Dave isn't big on exercise. About once every 3 years we take him to the doctors and have his pores surgically opened."

In this part . . .

You're going to push your body in familiar and not-so-familiar ways with stretches, speed drills, and weight exercises that target your muscular strength, flexibility, agility, coordination, and other fitness elements. Before you get started, however, we provide a few guidelines on technique and weight lifting to get you going. Once you get going, you'll relive those basic moves you learned long ago — only this time we emphasize proper form for injury prevention. Take it further with our simple and multimuscle moves. If you're in shape and following the Athletic Plan, you may want to try the power moves and skill drills.

Chapter 13

Technique, Technique, Technique

⬤ ⬤

In This Chapter

▶ Understanding why good form is important

▶ Learning the rules of proper technique

⬤ ⬤

*H*ow you perform an exercise or activity is as important as what kind of exercise you do. Because even if you're doing the best exercise in the world, if you do it with poor technique, it's going to be less effective and possibly even harmful. Either consequence ultimately causes you to stop exercising, thereby halting any body-transforming results. So before we show you all the moves that we've included in our Cross-Training Plans, we want to emphasize how important it is to do them all with extreme precision and control — from the slowest and simplest exercise that you may have done a million times before, to the highest impact and most intense move that you might do on occasion to give your training a challenging turbocharge.

We provide you with approximately 75 exercises from which you can pick and choose for your Cross-Training Plan. The fabulous news is that all the exercises that we recommend will change your body, improve your fitness, and notch up your sports performance and skills several levels. When you do them with an extra emphasis on precision, you'll get even more body-boosting benefits including increased total body balance, control, and stability. This is great when it comes to the crunch in a sport and you need to be able to push it to that next level either by generating a little more power, cranking out a little more speed, or lasting a few crucial minutes longer. When you focus on technique, you fine-tune your body. You'll not only be in fine fighting form, you'll be in superb fighting form.

This chapter introduces you to a few golden rules to keep in mind whenever you stretch, pump iron, or do sweaty drills on the field.

Why Poor Form Doesn't Cut It

Bad technique can lead to injuries. Good technique all boils down to doing something well as opposed to sloppy. To perform an exercise well, you need to concentrate — even though it's easy to get distracted. It's pretty obvious to our critical exercise-eyes when a client we train or a student in a class isn't paying attention to his movement. It could be something as simple as a vague look of boredom in his eyes or moving with a little too much speed to perform the exercise with a sufficient amount of muscular effort. In some cases it's pretty blatant, like when someone is watching TV while they work out. How can you pay any attention to your technique if you're caught up in the drama of *Law and Order*?

Sometimes even if you think you're doing an exercise carefully, you can still have bad form. You could be doing a push-up and trying to keep your spine in a straight line but be locking your elbows every time you come up. Or you could be performing a squat, trying to focus on squeezing the glutes but not realizing that your knees are jutting too far forward past your toes. We both feel that the most common mishap when it comes to form — no matter the exercise — is poor spinal posture. And it looks like night and day when you do a move correctly.

You'll look thinner, taller, more confident, and more attractive when you stand and sit up straight (plus your tummy will look flatter). Good posture also helps improve your skill level, strength, breathing, and ability to push your body to do great things because a properly aligned spine enables all your muscles to work more smoothly together.

Case study: Proper technique pays off

Tony's new client was in good shape and wanted to be pushed to the next level. John had been on a serious weight lifting program and had gained 15 pounds of muscle mass — going from wimp to wow in just six months. Tony noticed that as strong as John was, he couldn't do basic movements like pull his shoulder blades together. During the first session, Tony took out all the tough stuff and went over simple movement patterns and posture and flexibility exercises. John became noticeably frustrated and said he could handle more of a workout than these easy moves. When he left the session, he went to another gym to get a harder workout. During his next session with Tony, Tony explained to him that if he was more concerned about brute strength and pushing himself to the limits before he was able to execute basic moves properly then he might as well forget exercises, all he had to do was drag an anchor around all day. He persuaded John to rethink his priorities and give focusing on the *quality* of his movement a try. Tony put him on a program to perfect basic skills. The precision paid off. Eventually, John went on to do intense obstacle courses, plyometric moves, and Olympic lifts (weight lifting moves) — only this time stronger, with better posture, and injury-free.

The Rules of the Game

Poor form can have many causes, so we've put our heads together to pin-point the most common problems we've seen. So that you get the most out of all your moves, we've put together an easy list of key technique tips. Ignore them at your own peril!

Stop the slump

Whatever you do, we want you to keep a saggy spine out of it. The problem is that most of us are used to being in bad posture most of the time. Whether you hump over at your desk for many hours a day, slouch into the couch during TV time, or slump while you wait in line at the grocery store, you're probably stuck in bad back habits. Unfortunately, the more minutes and hours and months you hold the wrong back position, the more permanent it becomes. Poor spinal posture can result in one or a combination of the following:

✔ A slumped spine

✔ An overarched back or neck

✔ Rounded shoulders

✔ An extreme pelvic tilt

✔ A lopsided lean in one direction

The irony is this: Poor posture doesn't always mean that your back muscles are weak. In fact, they could be fairly strong, but they're strong in the wrong position. They're perfectly capable of supporting your spine in your slouch, but the minute you try to stand up straight for any period of time they get tired and it becomes uncomfortable. Betcha didn't know that sitting and standing up straight is actually an exercise? Our advice? Do it as much as you can, whenever you remember, whatever you happen to be doing.

We have to tell you the truth: A few back exercises during your weekly work-outs won't counteract the hours you spend standing or sitting the crooked way. So even though we have some great back-strengthening moves for you, you're going to have to do a little more to significantly improve your overall posture. The first step is to hold perfect posture during every exercise, not just those working your back.

If you're already a slouch potato, you'll probably remain one while you exercise, so take special notice of our alignment tips and cues to help you perfect your posture. Even if you're strong and you seem to be able to hold good form, don't think you're immune. Because once your muscles get fatigued, you get distracted. Even if you're concentrating so hard on one part of your body that you forget everything else, you can easily slip into a slump. The body likes to take the path of least resistance, so it's always prone to leaning and swaying to compensate for weaker body parts. Letting the stronger bits do most of the work can lead to chronic weakness or muscle imbalances in your body.

Your spine is an elegant structure consisting of a stack of roughly 32 building blocks — except, these *vertebrae,* as they're collectively called, are more like the leaning tower of Pisa. Your spine forms a subtle S-shape. Anything that curves to the extreme is considered poor form. "Standing up straight" is the posture that maintains your natural spinal curves. Good posture means standing with your head high, chin and head slightly forward, shoulders down and slightly back, chest and ribs lifted and pelvis in a neutral position, neither too far forward nor back.

Although most of us are familiar with the concept of good posture while standing and sitting, once you start to move, your spine and other skeletal bits get thrown in all different directions. So good posture can vary according to what you're doing. As a general rule, we want you to remember to elongate your spine in all positions. Some images we like to use as triggers to remind you how to hold yourself in good posture are

✔ Embrace your spine with your shoulder blades by moving your shoulders towards the back.

✔ Lift your rib cage away from your pelvis to lengthen the lower back.

✔ Pretend there's a string tied to the top of your head pulling you up and creating more space in between each segment of your spine.

✔ When you lean forward, keep your back straight and elongated, bending from the hips rather than the waist. Think of your spine as a diagonal arrow, from hips to head, lifting your torso as you lengthen.

The pelvic tilt

Many women have been conditioned to hold themselves in a spinal position that originated from dance techniques. This stance involves tilting the pelvis forward by pushing the buttocks forward so that the tailbone tilts down or to the front. This is intended to straighten out the lower back. In fact, a natural arch at the lower back is normal skeletal structure, and your back is strongest when you maintain this curve.

However, if you have an excessive arch in the lower back, a case could be made for holding it in a tilted position. Just as if your lower back was excessively rounded, it might be beneficial to tilt in reverse by pushing your bottom out in back. But for most of us, the pelvis should simply be centered; avoid adding pressure to the lower spine by flexing it and tilting it under.

✔ Drop scrunched-up shoulders by shrugging your shoulders to your ears, then letting them go.

✔ Lower your chin to avoid arching your neck. Look forward, rather than up.

Right Angle Rule

This is Tony's favorite rule, and the jist of it is this: Whenever you do an exercise, whether it's with your arms, your legs, or both, you'll be moving the limbs in different planes in both bent and straight positions. Since joints can get stressed at some angles, your chances of maintaining proper form for most exercises are best if you think _ninety degrees of separation._

When you raise your arm in front, stop at shoulder level (see that 90 degree angle between your upper arm and torso?). When you bend your knees in a squat position, keep your calves perpendicular to the floor so that your knees stop just before your toes and your body weight is held in the heel, not the ball of your foot. Your back is straight but leaning slightly forward (see those 90 degree angles at the knee, hip, and ankle joints?). This rule applies to almost any standing bent-knee position (squats, lunges, jumps, pliés, and so on). See Figure 13-1.

The general idea is to keep your limbs stacked evenly and as many body parts as possible parallel. The joints involved in each movement are likely to be held in their strongest, most stable position here. Now this doesn't mean that during certain phases of certain exercises you shouldn't move a joint into a smaller or bigger range of motion. Sometimes a more extreme angle is required and perfectly safe. But this is a visual trigger that you can use to monitor your body, especially when you're performing a move where you're unsure of the right positioning. So when in doubt, scout that square out.

Breathe smoothly

Okay, this seems as obvious as telling your heart to beat, but you'd be surprised at how many people hold their breath without realizing it. If you're really concentrating on squeezing your muscle during a particular strength exercise, or you find yourself in a position that requires a higher degree of control (balancing on one leg while manipulating the other leg), you might hold your breath as a reflex when trying to control your body.

Some moves that employ abdominal contractions might cause you to work with your diaphragm muscles, which can in turn inhibit your breathing. Sometimes just using a heavier-than-usual weight during an exercise encourages you to subconsciously alter your breathing pattern in an attempt to exert the force to move the weight.

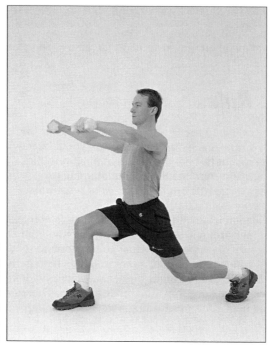

Figure 13-1:
Admire and
count all the
right angles
in this lunge.

Of course, there's the opposite extreme. Some people are so intent on breathing right that they force their breathing into an unnatural pattern — often ending up making loud, short, fast breaths and hyperventilating in the process.

Remember these three keys to breathing:

- **You should breathe according to your individual lung capacity.** Inhale and exhale fully, making each phase of your breath long, deep, and satisfying (like sex). The fitter you are and the bigger you are, the slower and longer your breaths will be because you have a larger lung capacity.

- **You should exhale on the effort during strength moves.** Some gym rats make a big show when they pump iron. They grunt, groan, grimace, and make all sorts of comedic gestures so that everyone will notice how strong they are. We think this is a sign that they're either lifting more weight than they can handle, or worse, they're creating a dangerous breathing pattern.

    The heavier your weight is (and this applies even if you're just using body weight), the more carefully you should make sure that you breathe out when you're exerting the most force with your body. This helps prevent a nasty physical reaction called the *Valsalva maneuver,* which occurs when you hold your breath by blocking the flow of air through your throat. An increase in internal body pressure can cause changes in blood pressure to worrying levels. The way to prevent this is to breathe regularly and exhale on the exertion. Make it look easy, for goodness sake. Relaxing your face to smile can also help release some of that pent-up air.

✔ ***Don't* stifle your breathing patterns during faster activities.** Whether it's a cardiovascular run or basketball game, a plyometric jump or a series of speed sprints between cones, don't worry about your breath too much. Just breathe naturally, regularly, and deeply so you can get all the energy-infusing oxygen into the muscles that need it.

Many people inhale through their nose and exhale from their mouth, except at higher intensities of exercise where it may all come from the mouth. No research is available that shows that any one method is better than any other, and chances are, you'll fall into the pattern that's most comfortable for you. Generally, the lower intensity the exercise is (a simple squat or ab crunch), you'll be more likely to use your nose. The more aerobic your exercise is, the more likely you are to use your mouth and nose together to get a bigger supply of air in and out. Remember your mouth and nose are the doors to all that relaxing, empowering, and rejuvenating air. Open them.

Know your limits

Listen to your body and know when to progress or slow down according to what you hear. Your body will give you signals to tell you what it needs. As you get more in touch and in control of your body and all it can do, these messages will become clearer. You'll know to cut out a particular jump if you are aware that it produces too much stress on your knees. Or you'll know when to ease off from a deep stretch that hurts more than helps.

A classic example of how listening to your body while you move can help you determine what's right for you is one of the old-school exercises everyone used to do for their abs. The lying double leg lift was a move that, while lying down, you lifted both legs two to six inches off the ground. Some variations placed your hands underneath your bottom, some versions had you lift your legs from the floor all the way up to a vertical position and then back down again. In sports circles, this move has always had the reputation as being one of the toughest, most advanced ab moves you could do. (This assumption was based on the fact that it is pretty painful to do.) In fact, if you analyze where the pain is coming from, you'd find that it stems from all the pressure in the lower back. The abs don't do much work at all since it's the hip flexor muscles that actually move the legs up and down. It's one of those moves that feels like it's doing one thing, but actually it's doing another. And in truth, it doesn't fatigue the abdominal muscles much at all, and is pretty stressful to the back. So to assess what's right for you, remember: Whenever you work out, focus inwards on all the good (and bad) sensations you feel.

Quality over quantity

Much of our society wants more, more, more (and Martica says that in her native Texas the ethos that "more is more" is especially true, particularly when it comes to jewelry, clothes, makeup, and hair volume). So it's not surprising that we carry that belief into the gym. The most strident example of this is the thousands of ab crunches so many regular exercisers pride themselves on being able to do. Some people do hundreds of repetitions of ab exercises a day. Multiple repetitions equals endurance training, not strength training. If you want strong, rippled muscles, getting stronger, rather than lasting longer, is the most effective way to do it.

So when you see someone hard at work on her gazillionth ab curl, this is something to keep in mind. Just because she can do that many doesn't mean she should, and just because she is doesn't mean she's getting stronger, more sculpted abs. In fact, one study found that subjects who were able to do high numbers of repetitions of abdominal moves actually had very little abdominal strength. The moral of the story: More is not better.

Another version of this principle is sometimes when you exercise — once fatigue, boredom, or distraction set in — you lose sight of the quality of your movement. It might happen when you're doing a series of cone sprints and you're so tired that you're stopping improperly and putting strain on your knees. Or it might happen when you're doing a set of sloppy squats. In all cases, it's better to slow down, back up, and re-establish control. Don't worry about finishing the exact number of repetitions. Do what you can, as perfectly as possible.

Feel like a feather

The better shape you're in, the more you can push your body to the next level. Ultimately this means going faster, harder, and longer — often adding more impact into your workouts. Since pushing it, by definition, means adding more stress to the joints, make sure that you still maintain control over your body no matter how high the intensity of your workout is. When you land, whether it's after a jump, after a running step, or when you're simply taking the next leg forward in a walking lunge, act like a feather. Land softly. Imagine keeping your body raised and lifted throughout all your activities. Keep your body light so that all the moves you do are less jarring to your joints. If this seems like an easy way out, it's not. In fact, your goal during any sport or exercise program is to make what might be an incredibly intense move look effortless. Picture the graceful leap of a ballet dancer (no mean feat). Notice what looks like a floating sprint down the field or an almost gentle catch at the goal line in a world-class football touchdown.

Avoid extremes

When it comes to moves, *hyper* means moving into a more extreme range of motion. When you squat low on your haunches, your knees are in hyperflexion (no right angle here). When you're doing a gymnastic back bend, your back is in severe hyperextension. Hyperextension or hyperflexion can apply to all your joints and if you're not strong enough to control your movement or flexible enough to bend that far, you probably should avoid bringing a joint into these ranges — especially when doing an exercise with weight, at speed, or in a loaded position (supporting your body weight). There will be some instances when you do want to move at the ends of your range of motion. Many sports movements require that you do so, especially in gymnastics, swimming, and running hurdles. And sometimes, if your joint has been held for prolonged periods in one position, it's good to reverse the position. For example, if you slump forward over a desk all day, the modified Cobra stretch — where you lie on your stomach and lean on your bent elbows — can help release the forward-bending stress on the spine. Just like the Right Angle Rule, you'll notice some instances when you may need to hyperflex or hyperextend, but for most purposes, stay within more moderate ranges of motion.

Burn, baby, burn?

Do you remember back in the early days of aerobics in the early 1980s? A typical Jane Fonda-style move was to stand in place with your arms outstretched to the sides, while you make zillions of tiny little circles with your hands. The men laughed at this wimpy arm exercise. But to the women doing it, they felt a hefty burn, which meant that surely it was working.

In fact, the exercise did fatigue the shoulder muscles for reasons that we won't go into too much here. (Okay, if you're curious, it's essentially because they were holding their arms up in an isometric contraction for an extended period of time and accumulating a buildup of lactic acid.) But these moves didn't produce the strong sculpted shoulders that exercising women have today. That's because the multiple shoulder circles were simply building up endurance or the ability to do more and more circles. Physiologically they weren't causing significant changes in strength, muscle mass, or muscle firmness. Once women learned that picking up a dumbbell and doing three sets of 12 lateral arm raises would give them a much stronger and shapelier shoulder, they could drop that old arm exercise which, by most accounts, was simply a waste of time.

Maintain control

The success of your workouts (that is, the results you get) depends upon how well you execute the exercises. An exercise is the sum of all the parts involved, and it's important to pay careful attention from the starting position to the end and to all the movement in between. This way you'll be aware of all the shifts in alignment, body weight, and muscle action that take place. We give you precise instruction for each exercise we suggest. In fact, our exercise cues are almost as good as having a personal training session from one of us in person. So don't just look at the pictures and mimic what you see. Learn and appreciate how your body moves in and out of each position. With that understanding you'll gain control. And control is what it's all about when it comes to fine-tuning your body to its utmost physical capabilities.

Focus on what's happening

Realize that your body is a computer. Your nerves, brain, and muscles work together to program your body how to move. When you perform a new movement pattern — whether this is a new activity or type of exercise you're taking up, or it's just better and more perfect form or skills you're trying to develop — establish the best possible way of moving that you can. Reprogram yourself. Exercise helps improve the messages between the brain and central nervous system to your muscles.

Break down each exercise to its finest points to get in touch with your body. Take inventory of all the muscles and actions that move you into each position.

Start each exercise slowly, focusing on the control part (perfect technique and alignment). Then and at the point of maximal contraction, such as when your elbow is bent in a biceps curl or you're in the stopping point of your lunge, focus on the *prime mover* muscle, the muscle or muscles that are holding you in that position. Disassociate yourself from all other body parts and try to elicit a maximal contraction or squeeze by focusing on the primary muscle or muscles involved. Relax everything else as much as possible. So, instead of gripping hard with a white knuckle grip during the biceps curl, relax your fists just enough to support the weight and then relax your head, neck, face, and jaw. Shift your attention back to the actual biceps. Pause for a second, then, as if you've just hit the Enter button, connect with that target muscle. At that moment you're at one with your muscle. The feeling here is effortless. This is a joining of mind and body.

Think strong thoughts

Okay, we want you to be safe, but we want you to challenge yourself too. Exercise is a fine line between putting the right amount of stress on your muscles, cardio and central nervous system to elicit positive physiological changes. So when you're nearing your last rep, focus on your working muscle and squeeze it harder. When you're coming into the finish of your walk or run, pick up the pace. If you feel like it, make it a sprint — even if that sprint is merely a faster walk. When you're getting ready to do another set of biceps curls, add a couple more pounds of weight or reset your focus to do the move with more perfect form.

But of course, it's not always this simple. Once you've achieved a certain level of fitness, it's easy to stay at status quo. Sometimes pushing yourself becomes harder mentally than it is physically. (Let's face it, who wouldn't prefer to slack off given the chance?) Tony likes to refer to this struggle as *actual output versus potential output*: potentially you could do more, but actually you won't. If you give yourself a little positive self-talk and think strong thoughts, you can work closer to your potential.

Mind tricks can help. If you're lifting a weight, try imagining that you're picking up or pushing something bigger, larger, and heavier. In fact, imagining yourself doing the impossible, such as tipping over a big Mack truck, might just trigger the extra few muscle fibers you're trying to challenge. Or if you're tired but trying to go that extra mile (or even that extra minute), relate what you're doing to something more practical. If you're on a cardio machine, imagine running with your baby (or soccer buddies), and feel the energy surge that you experience then. If you're on a long jog, focus on a distant point and imagine that it is a finish line. As you run, see it coming closer to you. You might just speed up without having to consciously make the effort to do so. Empower yourself to become more powerful.

Turn yourself on

Now that you know how to hold yourself and keep yourself aligned when you move, we want you to activate your body so you're primed for action. Trigger your postural muscles to sit up straight, turn on your brain to absorb all you're about to learn, and get ready to move!

Chapter 14

Your Weight Lifting Questions Answered

· ·

In This Chapter

▶ Dumbbells, rubber bands, and other ways to push your muscles

▶ Resistance training: How much, how often, how hard?

· ·

*I*t's one thing to know a little bit about how muscles work, it's another thing to know how to work them. We rounded up the most common questions that we've been asked by the people we've trained. You'll find out all the specifics, from what kind of resistance to use, to how often to do resistance training. Couple these practical tips with the savvy technique advice we give you in Chapter 13, and you'll be flaunting and flexing your curves in no time!

What Is Resistance Training?

Don't think you're a dumbbell if you've never been quite sure of what resistance training is. The term gets bandied about by the fitness savvy but can sound a little obscure if you're not quite sure what it refers to. Think taffy: Whether you push or pull, there's a little bit of a struggle because the tightness resists the movement. Resistance is simply an external force that makes your muscles work harder in order to move your body. It can be wind that you run against, a hill that you cycle up, water that you swim through, or a heavy weight that you lift. All forms of exercise, whether they are fast-moving activities like cycling or slow-moving exercises on a weight machine, involve some degree of resistance. *Resistance training,* however, refers to strength training exercise, usually done with some form of added weight like dumbbells or barbells.

Do I Have to Use Dumbbells?

The key to good results is using enough resistance to challenge your body. As long as you give your muscles the right push, any of the many resistance tools available will work. You'll never get bored because you can choose from many types of resistance! The most common are weight machines (as you would see in the gym), free weights (dumbbells and weighted bars), and elastic bands. Resistance doesn't have to be external, however. Your own body weight can act as resistance during some exercises, such as a push-up or squat. (One recent book suggested doing strength exercises with your cat, averaging around 10 pounds, not such a bad dumbbell, unless you count the claws!) You can also use mental focus to challenge the muscles to squeeze harder:

- **Weights:** Weights allow you to manipulate the amount you use very precisely. If one muscle group is weak, you can use lighter weights than you would when working a stronger muscle group. If a specific area in one muscle is weaker than other areas, you can perform part of the same exercise with a light weight and progress to a heavier weight in the range of motion that is stronger. You can train with weight machines or free weights.

  Weight machines are the big steel contraptions where you push or pull a weight stack that's attached to a pulley or chain (some machines have a form of hydraulics to provide resistance). They are great for beginners since they have a designated seat and handles. They are easy to use because you don't have to remember specific exercises; the machine automatically puts you in the proper position and leads you through each movement. The machines have handles positioned in a specific place (over your head, for example). You grab them and push or pull depending on the exercise. But because weight machines make you train in a specified position, they offer a limited selection of exercises that you can perform on them.

  Free weights, so-named because you can move them freely, are dumbbells and barbells that you hold in your hands. You get a much more functional workout because you can change the positions in which you do your exercises and you can call other muscles into action to help you balance the moving limb and stabilize the torso — something you won't do with weight machines. Although you do have to learn which exercises to do, once you're familiar with them, free weights are considered better all-round.

- **Elastic bands and rubber tubing:** To stretch these elastic fitness tools, your muscle must exert increasing levels of force to overcome the resistance. Although they look like a flimsy alternative, studies show that you can get similar strength gains to a traditional weight lifting workout.

They come in many shapes and strengths — colorful elastic strips or rubber tubes. Some look like big rubber bands, while others are long strips of plastic or surgical tubing with handles on each end. Bands are light, compact, and great for traveling. But they are sometimes more awkward to hold than a dumbbell or bar. Plus, you can't work all muscle groups in all positions very easily, and it's more difficult to control the tension in a band. When you use a weight, you can increase pound by pound; however, tension sizes of bands come in a limited range, so it might be difficult to control the progression of your exercises as precisely. When the band is too tight, it's difficult to complete the exercise from the starting to ending position. This means you train the muscle through only a small range of motion, which could lead to a weakness in certain degrees of movement around that joint. Still, they're a nice alternative to dumbbells at times, and you'll still find many fitness classes using them instead of, or along with, regular weights.

✔ **Body weight exercise:** Moving while supporting your own body weight is also an effective form of resistance. You can add more or less resistance to an exercise by manipulating how much weight the limb you're working must support. For example, if you stand and then bend and straighten your leg in an exercise squat, your muscles will work much harder than if you bend and straighten your legs while lying down. Push-ups require that you support a lot of body weight. The only problem with using your body as resistance is that you have a limited range of exercises you can do with this form of resistance, so for some muscle groups, you do need to use weights or bands.

✔ **Stability ball:** The latest resistance tool that's taken the exercise world by storm is the stability ball: a big, rubber ball that you sit, lie, or stand on while doing different exercises. Because it makes you unstable, your muscles work extra hard to stabilize your body. You can use the ball to stretch by wrapping different parts of your body around it in different positions. You can use it to do abdominal exercises, push-ups, pelvic tilts, and other strength moves. During ab moves, you can lean your body backward across the ball before you curl up, which is something you definitely can't do on the floor. This, plus the fact that you have to stabilize yourself to keep from wobbling, adds more resistance to your ab exercises.

✔ **Balance boards:** Balance boards operate on the skateboarding premise: hop onto something that makes you wobble, see how long you can last on it, and see what you can do while you're up there. You can choose from many types of balance boards, but generally they are a flat platform atop a round base. Your core torso and leg muscles work hard to keep you centered and stable. You can simply stand on one and try to balance (a great butt and ab workout); or to make things harder, you can do traditional strength exercises like biceps curls and arm raises while perched on one.

All types of resistance improve muscle strength and tone as long as you consistently provide adequate stimulus to the muscles you work.

How Often Should I Do Resistance Training?

The good news: Research shows that you shouldn't lift weights too often. Whereas you can do aerobic exercise daily, resistance exercises exhaust your muscles so much that they need time to recover. So for best results, lift weights every other day, two to three times a week.

Some people do perform resistance exercises every day; this is okay as long as you're working different muscle groups on consecutive days. If you have the time to train like this, split up the body parts you target on different days rather than do a total body routine each session. You might train your biceps and triceps on Monday, chest and legs on Tuesday, abs and back on Wednesday, and biceps and triceps on Thursday, and so on. Instead of doing just one exercise per muscle group, you might target the body part with several different moves in order to target the widest amount of muscle fibers.

How Much Weight Should I Lift?

The general rule is to use enough weight so that by the end of one set of about 8-12 repetitions your muscle feels tired. If you don't feel the weight getting heavy and the muscle fatiguing by the end of each set and if you feel like you could do more than a couple of reps, you're not stimulating the muscle enough to make it adapt and grow stronger. You need to use more resistance. If you can't complete eight repetitions because the weight is too heavy, you need to use less weight.

If you want to get technical, you can figure out the precise amount of weight you should use by going to the gym and determining how strong each muscle is. Your *repetition maximum* (RM) is the most weight you can lift for any given muscle at one time. If you choose a 20-pound weight, for example, and can do a biceps curl two times, this isn't your maximum. The amount of weight you could lift one time with good form represents how strong you are. (If you're a beginner, this test isn't a good idea because you may lift more weight than you're ready for.) Once you find your RM for each muscle group and individual exercise, you would then start training by working with 60-80 percent of the RM. So if 20 pounds is your RM for biceps curls, you could start with 12-16 pounds. This means that you should be able to complete a set of 8-12 repetitions before your muscle fatigues. However, getting this specific and finding out your RM is not really necessary. You can get a good estimate of how much to lift through trial and error.

Start with a light weight and work your way up. If you pick up a weight and feel strain in your joints right away, or if you can hardly move it, it's too heavy. If you can swing the weight around very easily, it's too light. Beginners — especially women — think they are much weaker than they really are. (Think of the 30-pound suitcase, 5-pound handbag, 10-pound laundry basket, and 15-pound grocery bag you haul around.) If you have been exercising fairly regularly, especially if you have used weights before, you don't necessarily need to start with an ultra-light 1-pound weight. You may try 2 or 5 pounds. You can always decrease the weight if you need to.

Because muscles come in many shapes and sizes — and some have been used more over the years than others — you'll find that some muscle groups are stronger than others. So it's a good idea to vary the amount of weight you use. You may be able to use quite heavy weights for your stronger biceps (front of the upper arm) and deltoids (shoulder), but very light ones for your weaker triceps (back of the upper arm) or trapezius (upper back). If you use a lighter weight for a strong muscle, you might not challenge it sufficiently to make it stronger; if you use a weight that's too heavy for a smaller, weaker muscle, you might not be able to complete the number of repetitions required and could strain the joint.

How Many Repetitions of an Exercise Should I Do?

When you first do *any* exercise, you'll experience *slight* gains in strength. But if the exercise doesn't become progressively more challenging, your strength ceases to increase. So you may need to do more and more repetitions to feel fatigued. However, a fine line exists between strength and endurance. Doing more and more reps may feel like you're fatiguing the muscles, but you may only be targeting the endurance, slow-twitch fibers (see Chapter 7). You may feel a burning sensation, but this is simply a buildup of waste products in an area caused by holding a body part in a set position and repeating a movement over and over. This is not true fatigue caused from working the muscle to exertion. To get stronger and firmer, you need to overload by challenging the muscle to exert more force, *not* to exert the same amount of force for a longer period.

If you're training for strength, fatigue your muscles within 30-90 seconds of performing an exercise. Studies show that working a specific muscle any longer than this means you focus more on developing endurance. For most people, this means using about 75 percent of the maximum force a muscle can exert, or 75 percent of RM (see the "How Much Weight Should I Lift?" section), and doing 8-12 repetitions of an exercise.

At the end of each set of repetitions, you should feel muscular fatigue, which shows you're challenging your muscles to exert enough force so that they tire out. You might not feel a burning sensation, only weakness, and your muscles may quiver. This will trigger the muscles to recover and get stronger. If you feel nothing at the end of a set of exercises, chances are you haven't challenged the muscles enough, and you will only maintain, not improve upon, your current levels of strength. If you continue on by doing more repetitions, you'll switch the training emphasis to endurance rather than strength.

How Many Sets Should I Do?

One set is a group of repetitions. The traditional training formula is one to three sets of 8-12 repetitions of each exercise. Some bodybuilders and athletes may do five sets or more of each exercise. Studies show that most of the increases in strength come from doing one set of 8-12 reps. Additional sets contribute to further improvements, but as long as you're executing the moves properly and with a challenging amount of resistance, you don't have to do more to get great results.

How Fast Should I Lift Weights?

Since you cut out the help of momentum, going slower generally makes you work a little harder. Slower weight training is good for beginners or if you're trying out new exercises because you can also monitor your body alignment and technique more easily. Move the weight in each direction for a count of two to four (one, two, three, four, pause. One, two, three, four, pause). Hold the position for a second before changing directions to stop the momentum and focus on your alignment. Concentrate on going a little slower during the return phase. Consciously resist against the reflex to swing back or drop down to your starting position.

Moving weights quickly is a power training tool — a good technique to incorporate if you're strong enough to execute the movements with control.

How fast you move on to another exercise or the next set affects the intensity — and results — of your workout. For best results, wait no more than 90 seconds in between sets. *Circuit training,* a weight workout where you move quickly from one weight exercise to another, employs this method. This is an invigorating workout, but it's very tough. If you're new or trying out new exercises, keep it slow.

Chapter 15

Warm-ups and Stretches

In This Chapter

▶ Why warm is better

▶ Cooling down from a vigorous workout

▶ What stretching can (and can't do)

*B*efore you launch into the tuff stuff, you need to prepare your body. This chapter explains why you need to ease into — and get out of — an intense workout slowly. We show you a wide range of stretches that target all the major muscles you'll be using during your workouts. Your body will respond better to exercise if you warm up first. Although there's no definitive proof to show that regular stretching definitely prevents injuries, most fitness trainers believe that a warmed up, flexible body will cope better with the demands of exercise. Plus, stretching feels fabulous!

Warming Up

We know you're just dying to jump straight into your new cross-training program with full force. But we want you to chill out for a minute, or rather, get warm. It's important to warm up slowly rather than plunge into a vigorous exercise session. By doing gentle exercise before you push yourself hard, your joints will become lubricated, you'll speed up your blood circulation, and you'll kickstart all the metabolic machinery in your body that helps you produce energy. A proper workout will help your body function as efficiently as possible during more vigorous exercise sessions, and you're more likely to last longer in the overall workout if you spend a little more time warming up.

You can warm up in a number of ways. Generally, the easiest thing to do is to start your chosen activity very slowly. If you're going to run, warm up with a walk for at least five minutes. If you're going to bike, warm up by cycling very slowly for five minutes or more. If you're playing a sport or taking a fitness class, your warm-up could be as simple as marching in place and walking while simulating some of the arm movements you'll use in the activity later on (biceps curls, arm raises, and so on). However you warm up, try to use all four limbs to prime them for action and keep it easy for 5–10 minutes.

Cooling Down

Slow down gradually after an intense cardio exercise like running or playing a sport. Stopping abruptly slows the clearance of lactic acid from the muscles. You can also become dizzy if you stop too suddenly. Slow the movements down until your heart rate returns to normal, or about 100 beats per minute. (Hint: if you're panting or gasping for breath, you're not ready to stop. Keep cooling down!) You might be interested to know that the fitter you are, the faster your body readjusts and your heart rate gets back to normal. To cool down, keep moving with a low-intensity version of your exercise for at least five minutes. If you are a beginner, or have done a particularly intense session, cool down for about 10 minutes. Since your body is warm, this is always a good time to sneak in your stretches. A proper cooldown and stretch should make you feel relaxed and energized.

Stretching Out

For some people *stretch* is synonymous with *ouch!* But it doesn't have to be that way. To those who don't stretch properly, it's a painful but necessary evil. To those who have discovered the secrets of elongating a muscle to its comfortable limits, stretching is a luxury that can induce palpable waves of pleasure (some say, almost like an orgasm) up and down a tight muscle. Don't believe it? Read on.

First of all, stretching is simply the movement you do to make your joints and muscles around them more flexible. There have been all sorts of fantastic claims about the miracle effects of stretching. It's said not only to prevent and/or cure injuries and soreness, but to make you longer, stronger, leaner, and taller. From what research tells us, not one of these assertions is a fact. However, stretching does have proven benefits. The more flexible you are, the more smoothly and easily your body will move, and the less stiff and tight you'll feel. A good stretch releases lots of muscle tension. This de-stressing effect will definitely make both your body and your mind feel more relaxed.

You can stretch in many ways. The simplest approach is what we call *sneak-a-stretch*. All you need to do is position your body in such a way that a particular muscle lengthens. So if you're at work and your legs have been scrunched up, sitting in a chair all day, you just need to put your leg straight out in front of you, propped up on a wastebasket or other chair if you can, and lean toward it slightly. You'll feel the hamstrings in the back thigh loosen up. One thing to keep in mind if you sneak-a-stretch is to keep the stretch small. Don't try to turn yourself into Gumby, because, since you're probably not warmed up, you may be more likely to pull too hard. Keep it slow and easy.

Pushing past your limits

If you exert force to stretch (yank your leg and grip tightly with your hands to pull a muscle harder), your muscles will respond by tightening, not relaxing. This is known as the *stretch reflex*. Sensors in the muscle fibers detect when a muscle is being pushed past its available range of motion. A signal is given for the muscle to contract, or shorten. Ironically, this is just when you're trying to lengthen it. If you continue to push past this tightness, the stretch becomes painful because you're causing microtears to the muscle cells. Ultimately, this leads to greater inflexibility, so don't push it. Stretching is about relaxation. The calmer your approach, the more flexible you will become. A contracted muscle won't stretch, so relax!

Getting stretchy

When it comes to the different stretching techniques, the most common is *static* stretching where you simply elongate your target muscle and hold it gently without moving until you feel it relax. *Ballistic stretching* is static stretching with a bounce. This can be quite painful since the whole idea is to force the muscle to stretch by pushing and pulling it into submission. Aerobics in the early 1980s famously used a "pulse" during assorted stretches to bounce into a deeper stretch. Many athletes and dancers who use their traditional training techniques still use it today, although we now know that ballistic stretching can strain a muscle because the bounce can elicit the opposite reaction. Rather than stretching and relaxing, the muscle tightens to protect itself from overstretching.

Other approaches like *Proprioceptive Neuromuscular Facilitation* (or PNF for those in the know*), Active Isolated stretching,* and *Contract, Relax, and Contract,* have you alternate muscle squeezes with muscle stretches to try to trigger the target muscle to relax even more. *Dynamic stretching* is simply when a muscle stretches while it is moving. Stretching in a tennis serve or while kicking a ball are examples of dynamic stretching. If you try to increase your flexibility this way, you have a good chance of pulling something because the dynamic part of the stretch means that you're exerting a lot of force along with momentum, allowing you little control if you stretch too far. When you perform movements that involve a dynamic stretch, it's better to keep your range of motion within your natural range of flexibility and try to improve your flexibility with one of the more effective and safe techniques.

If you're feeling experimental and want to apply the principle of cross-training to your stretching, this is how each method works:

✔ **Static:** Position yourself in a way that you are lengthening a desired muscle and hold for 10-30 seconds. If you feel pain, back up. Avoid forcing the muscle to do anything it clearly doesn't want to do. Relax, and then repeat at least 4 times.

✔ **Ballistic:** A static stretch with a bounce, pulse, or jerk. This is probably not the most effective approach.

✔ **Proprioceptive Neuromuscular Facilitation (PNF) stretching:** Contract the muscle you wish to stretch, and then relax and immediately stretch it, holding it for about 10 seconds. The idea is that by squeezing the muscle first, it will be doubly relaxed and become better able to stretch.

✔ **Active Isolated (AI):** Most muscles work in pairs, that is, an opposing muscle group helps move a shared joint in the opposite direction. So, when your biceps contract, they bend your elbow joint. At the same time, the triceps relax, or stretch. When the elbow straightens, the biceps relax and the triceps contract. To try Active Isolated stretching, contract the muscle opposite from the one you're trying to stretch and then immediately stretch the desired muscle, holding it for just a few seconds and repeating this switch-off up to 20 times.

✔ **Contract, Relax, and Contract (CRAC):** Here you complicate the process by first stretching your target muscle, then tightening your target muscle, then tightening its opposing muscle to relax the target muscle. Each phase is held for about 10 seconds.

✔ **Dynamic:** Using swinging and reaching movements to increase the range of motion around a joint, keep the movements small to prevent over-stretching.

We've kept it simple by providing a series of static stretches for you to do, both in this chapter and in Chapter 28. Some of the exercises and drills in Part IV also incorporate some dynamic flexibility within the movements.

Weight lifting has always gotten a bad rap when it comes to flexibility. People assumed that because it makes you strong, it makes you stiff. But this just isn't so. As long as you are doing exercises where you move your muscles in their full ranges of motion, you can actually improve your flexibility from weight lifting.

The American College of Sports Medicine recommends that you do flexibility exercises at least two or three days a week. You can either do all your stretching in one longer session, or include stretches at the start and end of your workouts. Your tissues are more easily stretched when they are warm. So always stretch after you have finished warm-up exercises or after a workout.

Stretch do's and don'ts

People tend to think that vigorous kinds of exercise like running and jumping are unsafe, while slow-moving activities like stretching and yoga are safe. This isn't necessarily the case. It's easy to overstretch if you push too far. You can become too flexible. Some yoga positions where you twist your body into pretzel-like poses, forcing body parts into unnatural positions, can not only strain muscles and tendons but they can cause long term damage to the ligaments and joints. People spend years trying to develop enough flexibility to achieve some of these poses, but they also end up overstretching their ligaments in the process. Ligaments support the joints they surround; if they get overstretched, they lengthen and the joint is permanently unstable, leaving it more susceptible to injury.

Then again, there are lots of super-tight, ultra-stiff, inflexible people out there who only stretch to reach for the remote control. These people need to stretch as much as they can. So that you can shoot for a body that's a happy medium between rigid and flimsy, we provide the key technique tips you should keep in mind when stretching:

✔ Avoid bouncing or forcing your body to stretch. Instead, hold a stretch gently, and do not pulse.

✔ Start with an easy, rather than a deep, stretch.

✔ If you feel any pain whatsoever, that's a sign that you've pushed yourself too far. Back up.

✔ Stretch enough so you feel pleasurable waves of tension release, not strain.

✔ Hold each stretch for 10–60 seconds. You can break up a prolonged stretch by alternating a stretch and release.

✔ Deep breathing helps release tension. Exhale as you elongate a muscle to help it lengthen and relax.

Total Body Stretches

Here are moves to stretch all your major muscle groups. We also include a chapter of stretches that you can do on a bench or your bed in Chapter 28. We provide a variety of stretches, some that work similar muscle groups in slightly different positions. You should experiment with all the stretches and use the ones that feel the most comfortable for your body.

Standing hip lunge stretch

Walking or climbing a lot of stairs can make your hip flexors tight. You'll use them even more during your workouts. Target these tight muscles in the front of your hips and thighs with this simple move.

Where You Feel It: Front of the back hip.

1. **Stand with your feet hip-width apart and parallel. Step forward with your left leg so that you are in a split-leg position. Hands are on your front thigh.**

2. **Step back with your right foot as far as you can and lower your hips until the front knee is bent to a 90 degree angle.**

3. **Press your right hip forward to feel the stretch in your right hip. Keep your back leg straight behind you and balance on your back toe, keeping your back heel off the ground. Once you feel flexible enough, lower your body so that your back leg rests on the ground with your knee down and the top of the foot resting on the floor (see Figure 15-1). Hold, and then switch legs.**

Safety Tip: If the stretch is too extreme on your hip, raise your body higher.

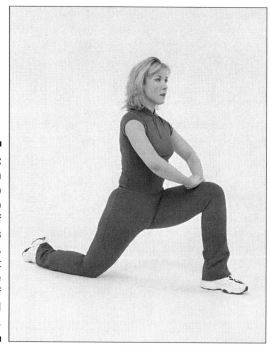

Figure 15-1:
This stretch will help loosen up the front of your hips and thighs, areas that get tense from lots of walking and sitting.

Standing hamstring and calf stretch

When the back of your thighs get tight, your lower back might arch slightly to compensate, and the way you hold yourself can shift to put more pressure on your spine.

Where You Feel It: Back of the front leg.

1. **Standing in a split leg position — right foot in front and left in back — bend your back left knee slightly and lean your upper body forward as you support your hands on the bent thigh.**

2. **Keep the right leg straight in front and push your right buttock out behind to stretch the front of the back thigh.**

3. **Lift your right toe up and then turn it inward so the bottom of your foot faces left. This will sneak in a little ankle stretch. In the same position, flex your right foot to move the stretch a little lower from the back of your thigh down to the calf (see Figure 15-2). Then switch sides.**

Where You Feel It: The calf of the front leg.

Safety Tip: If your calf hurts, bend your knee slightly and lower your front foot.

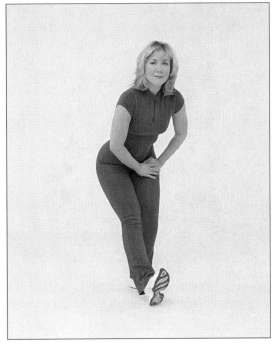

Figure 15-2:
Lower your toe if the stretch feels too intense in the back of your leg.

Seated hamstring stretch

You can target the back of the thighs even when you are sitting down watching TV by extending them and simply leaning forward.

Where You Feel It: The back of your legs.

1. **Sit with both legs extended in front of you. Place your hands by your sides.**

2. **Lift your rib cage and lean slightly forward to press your chest toward your thighs.**

3. **Hold and feel the back of your legs start to relax. Lower your shoulders and exhale to release the tension (see Figure 15-3).**

Safety Tip: If your lower back feels strained, lift your upper body and lean with a straight back at a slight diagonal forward; do not bend over.

Figure 15-3: Raise your upper body to decrease the hamstring stretch.

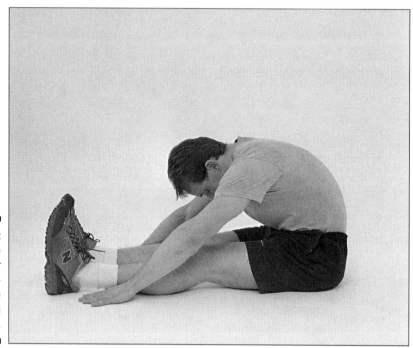

Glute and thigh stretch

A simple shift of your upper body is all you need to target two different muscle groups in this stretch (see Figure 15-4).

Where You Feel It: Gluteals of the front leg and quadriceps.

1. **Sit on the floor with your arms by your sides, palms flat. Bend your left knee in front of your body, knee bent to about 90 degrees.**

2. **Bend your right leg behind you so that your right foot aims toward the back. Lift the right heel off the ground slightly. This knee should be bent to about 90 degrees as well.**

3. **Lean your upper body back and slightly away from your right thigh to feel the stretch in the quadriceps, the front of the right thigh.**

4. **Then lean your torso forward over the top of your left thigh. Support your upper body weight by resting on your forearms. You'll feel the stretch here in the buttock of your left leg.**

Figure 15-4:
Lean back to feel the stretch in the quads, and then lean forward to feel it in the glutes.

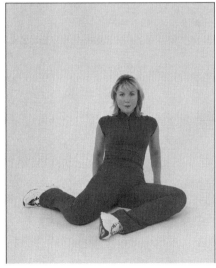
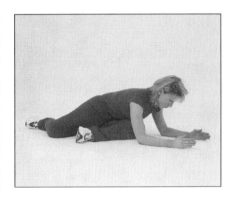

Wall pelvic tilt

You may want to increase the mobility of your lower back. This pelvic tilt stretches the lower portion of your spine.

Where You Feel It: Lower back.

1. **Stand facing a wall with your arms outstretched, hands at chest level pushing on the wall.**

2. **Walk your feet back so that your upper body is leaning slightly forward.**

3. **Pull your lower abs in and tilt your pelvis forward to round the lower back (see Figure 15-5).**

Safety Tip: If this strains your back, decrease the tilt of your pelvis.

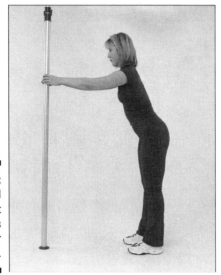 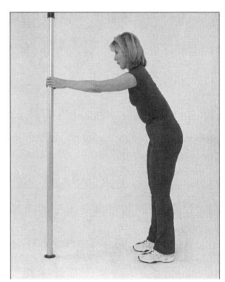

Figure 15-5:
The wall pelvic tilt stretches your lower back.

Calf and soleus stretch

Your lower legs support you when you stand, walk, and run. Try this stretch to increase the flexibility in this area.

Where You Feel It: Lower leg.

1. **Stand in front of a wall with your arms outstretched in front, hands flat against the wall. You can also grab a pole or pillar for support.**

2. **Step with your left toes on a dumbbell (or use a book if the dumbbell is on a smooth surface and rolls) so that the toes are raised higher than your heel on the floor (see Figure 15-6). Keep your left knee straight.**

3. **Now bend your left knee slightly (refer to the second photo in Figure 15-6).**

Safety Tip: If this pulls too much on your Achilles tendon, decrease the stretch by lowering your toe.

Figure 15-6:
You can shift the emphasis from the gastrocnemius to your soleus muscles simply by bending your knee.

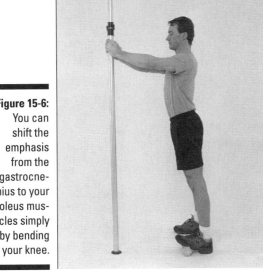
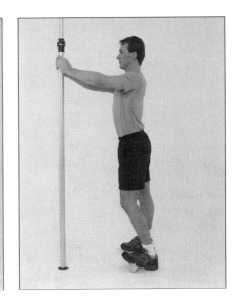

Foot and ankle stretch

Take off your shoes and give those tootsies a break! Your feet could be the most understretched muscles in your body. This stretch feels as good as a foot massage.

Where You Feel It: Top and bottom of foot.

1. **Take off your shoes. Stand with your feet hip-width apart, hands on your hips.**

2. **Bend your left knee slightly and raise your left foot and place the top of your foot down facing the floor slightly, just underneath your right hip but slightly behind your opposite ankle so that your toes curl slightly under. The bottom of your foot should face behind you, top of the foot presses down (see the left photo in Figure 15-7).**

3. **Now press the ball of your foot into the floor so that your toes flex and your heel lifts up. Press the bottom of your toes into the floor (see the right photo in Figure 15-7). Hold, and then switch feet.**

Safety Tip: When dropping your foot top down, if your toes cramp, move your foot farther behind so toes are not bent under.

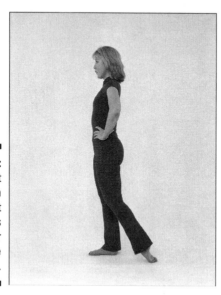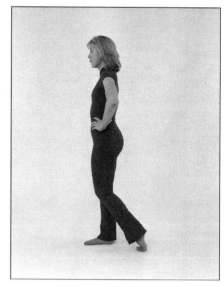

Figure 15-7: Identify tight spots in your foot and press into the floor to release the tension.

Lat stretch

If you carry tension in your back, you'll like this stretch that targets the big latissimus dorsi.

Where You Feel It: Across your back.

1. **Lean forward and grab onto a counter, pillar, or pole with your left arm.**

2. **Walk your feet back away from it until your arms are outstretched and your legs are in a split lunge position. Your right leg should be in front of the left, and the right knee should be bent to about 90 degrees.**

3. **Drop your head so your neck is in line with your spine and your body is in a flat back position.**

4. **Bend your knees slightly and push your hips back to pull away from the bar; open the shoulder blades and stretch out the back (see Figure 15-8).**

Safety Tip: If your shoulders feel strained from pulling, release some tension from your hand grip and focus on opening the shoulder blades and expanding your rib cage.

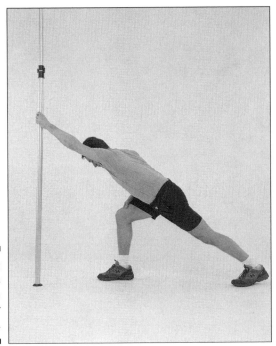

Figure 15-8:
Feel this
stretch
across your
back.

Deltoid and upper back

Where You Feel It: Back of your left shoulder and around the left shoulder blade.

1. **Stand next to a pole or a doorway sideways with your right shoulder next to it. Raise your left arm directly in front of your left shoulder and across your chest to hold onto the pole or door frame.**

2. **Keep your left hand at shoulder level (see Figure 15-9).**

3. **Rotate your chest slightly to the left.**

4. **Hold, and then switch sides.**

Safety Tip: Make sure your hand is rotated out so the palm faces the back wall, not down to the floor.

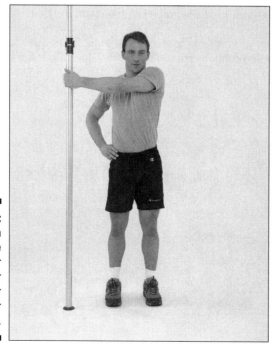

Figure 15-9:
This stretch targets the back of your shoulder and your shoulder blade.

Pectorals stretch

If you spend your days scrunched up over a desk, this chest stretch will help you release tight pectorals.

Where You Feel It: Upper inner arm and chest.

1. **Stand with your right side facing sideways to the doorway and grasp onto the corner with your right hand, palm against the wall.**

2. **Step far enough away from the wall that your arm is outstretched. Hand should be shoulder-level.**

3. **Turn your chest to the left (see Figure 15-10).**

4. **Raise your hand higher along the wall to head-level and again rotate your torso to the left.**

5. **Hold, and then switch arms.**

Safety Tip: If you feel any strain in your shoulder, decrease the range of motion of the stretch.

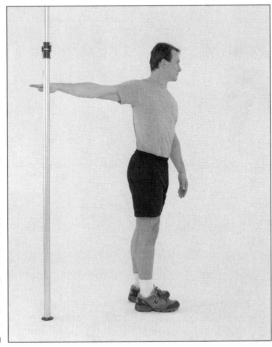

Figure 15-10:
Poor posture can lead to tight chest muscles. This stretch helps increase flexibility in the area.

Triceps stretch

You can target the back of your upper arms with this stretch.

Where You Feel It: Back of the upper arm and shoulder.

1. **Cross your right arm in front of your chest, hold onto the right elbow with the left hand, and raise the arm over your head. Pull the right elbow toward the left to feel the stretch in the upper arm.**

2. **Hold, and then switch sides (see Figure 15-11).**

Safety Tip: Raise arms slightly if you don't feel this in the upper arm.

Figure 15-11:
You'll feel this stretch in the back of your shoulders and the back of your upper arms.

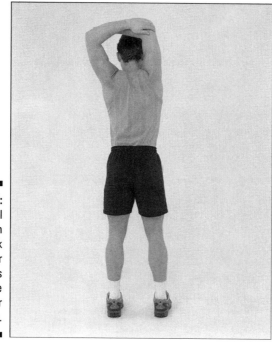

Biceps stretch

Open your chest and release the pent-up tension in your arms with this stretch.

Where You Feel It: Upper inner arms.

1. **Stand tall, spine elongated, ribs lifted away from the pelvis.**

2. **Open both arms in a T position out to the sides, pushing the arms slightly behind you and keeping hands at shoulder level, palms facing down.**

3. **Press your shoulders and the sides of your inner wrists forward to feel the stretch in the front of the upper arms (see Figure 15-12).**

Safety Tip: Avoid dropping your head back, and keep your chin level in front of your chest.

Figure 15-12: Try to push your biceps forward to increase this stretch.

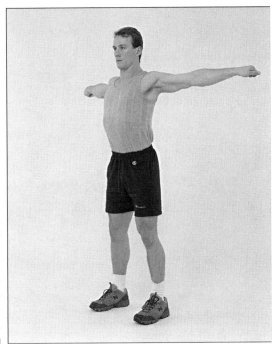

Neck stretch

The neck muscles can absorb a lot of tension during stressful or busy days. These moves will you loosen up.

Where You Feel It: Back and sides of the neck.

1. **While sitting, tilt your head to the right side with the right hand exerting a gentle pull sideways (see the left photo in Figure 15-13).**

2. **Hold, and then switch sides.**

3. **Remain sitting, and rest both hands on the back of your head. Drop your chin to your chest (see the right photo in Figure 15-13).**

Safety Tip: Don't pull on your head; simply let the weight hang to stretch the back of your neck.

Figure 15-13: Allow the weight of your head to drop, but avoid pressing down with your hands.

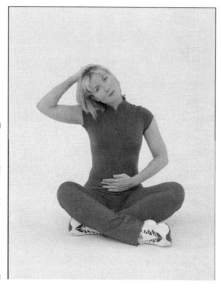 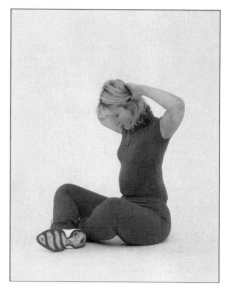

Chest stretch

Most of our daily lives are spent hunched forward: curled over a desk, slouched into a sofa, or slumped in our cars. To reverse the forward pressure on the spine, do this stretch to uncurl the back and stretch out your chest and front of the torso.

Where You Feel It: Front of your rib cage.

1. **Lie down on your stomach with your legs extended behind you.**

2. **Raise your chest and prop yourself up on your elbows.**

3. **Keep your chin level and look forward as you press your ribs to the front (see Figure 15-14).**

Safety Tip: If your lower back feels stressed, lower your chest slightly.

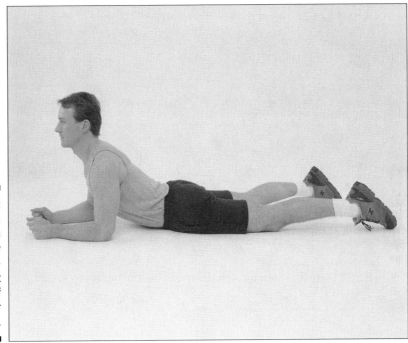

Figure 15-14:
This stretch reverses the daily forward-bent position of the lower back.

Back stretch

Open up your shoulder blades to relieve tightness in the upper back by rounding into this cat stretch.

Where You Feel It: Along entire back and in between the shoulder blades.

1. **Get on your hands and knees, and keep your back straight.**
2. **Press your chest to the floor, and then pull your bellybutton in.**
3. **Round your spine like a cat (see Figure 15-15).**

Safety Tip: If your lower back feels strained, decrease the curve of your back.

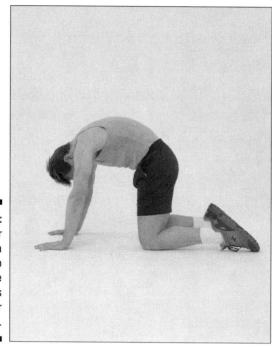

Figure 15-15:
Arch your back like a cat to stretch the muscles around your spine.

Upper back stretch

If you don't have a personal masseuse, this stretch may help target those hard-to-reach tight spots in the back.

Where You Feel It: Upper middle back.

1. **Get on your hands and knees on the floor. Slide your left arm forward on the floor, palm down, reaching over your head.**

2. **Reach your right arm under your body and through your left arm (see Figure 15-16).**

3. **Drop your chest to look through the left upper arm.**

4. **Open the shoulder blades to stretch the upper back.**

5. **Hold, and then switch sides.**

Safety Tip: If your knees feel uncomfortable, move your upper body farther forward.

Figure 15-16:
Place a pad underneath your knees and keep your hips raised if your knees feel uncomfortable during this upper back stretch.

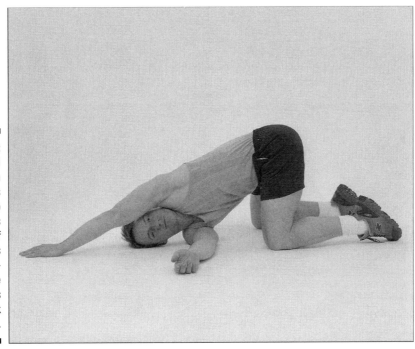

Side stretch

You can do this stretch standing or sitting, but try to lift up to elongate your spine as you lean to the side.

Where You Feel It: Side and back of torso.

1. **Sit cross-legged on the floor and grasp a rope, broom, or towel between both hands. Your hands should be shoulder-width apart.**

2. **Raise arms overhead with palms facing forward.**

3. **Lift your ribs to lengthen your spine as you lean slightly to left (see Figure 15-17).**

4. **Hold, and then switch sides.**

Safety Tip: If the stretch is too severe, place one hand on the floor next to you to support your upper body as you lean to the side.

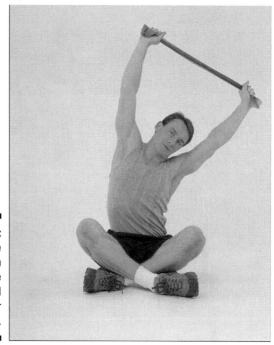

Figure 15-17: The side stretch works the side and back of your torso.

Spinal twist stretch

A gentle twist of the back can release tension in the back muscles that other stretches can't get to.

Where You Feel It: Back, buttocks, and chest.

1. **Lie on your back with your legs straight.**

2. **Open your arms into a T position out to the sides, palms down.**

3. **Cross your right leg over your left thigh so that your lower body twists in opposition to the stabilized upper body (see Figure 15-18). Look over your right shoulder.**

4. **Hold, and then switch sides.**

Safety Tip: If your feet can't rest comfortably on the floor, bend your knees slightly.

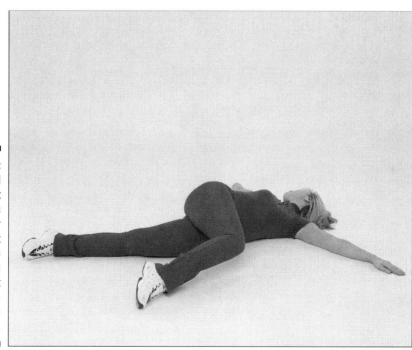

Figure 15-18: This spinal twist stretches the lower back, but you'll also feel it in your chest and buttocks of the top leg.

Chapter 16

Basic Moves Revisited

. . . .

In This Chapter

▶ Taking a new look at squats, plié squats, split lunges, back lunges, ab curls, reverse curls, push-ups, and triceps dips

▶ Mastering your movement skills

. . . .

*N*o doubt you're familiar with a lot of standard exercises such as squats, push-ups, ab curls, and lunges. But chances are, if you've spent a lifetime (or even a few months) doing them, you may have slipped into bad form habits — your knee might be just a tad too far forward in one move, and your back just a tiny bit misaligned in another. We want you to take a fresh look at these old moves. Spend time performing them, but instead of going on automatic pilot, pay special attention to our alignment points and technique tips. Then in the following chapters, you'll be ready to take on the more advanced moves, many of which use the standard positions in this chapter as their base.

We prescribe these, and the rest of the exercises in the upcoming chapters, to you in different groups and with different numbers of sets and reps, depending on the Cross-Training Plan you choose to follow (or devise yourself) in Part III. In general, however, whenever performing strength moves, do three sets of 8-12 repetitions. For best results, make sure you allow a day of rest in between working the same muscle groups.

Squat

This exercise (see Figure 16-1) is a very functional move. You squat every time you pick up luggage, kids, and grocery bags, as well as when you are in a neutral position, getting ready for the next play during many different sports.

Muscles worked: Gluteals, quadriceps, hamstrings, erector spinae, and abs.

1. **Stand tall with your feet parallel and hip-width apart. Hands should be holding dumbbells, hanging by your sides with your palms facing in.**

2. **With a straight back, lean your upper body slightly forward. At the same time, push your hips out behind you as you lower your pelvis into a sitting position. Stop when your thighs are almost parallel to the floor. Keep the knees bent to no less than a 90-degree angle.**

3. **Contract your glutes to squeeze back up to standing and repeat.**

Figure 16-1:
Squeeze your butt tight during both the lowering and lifting phases of this move.

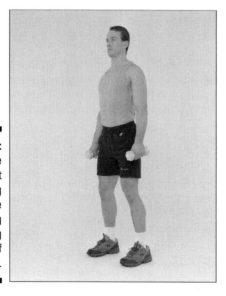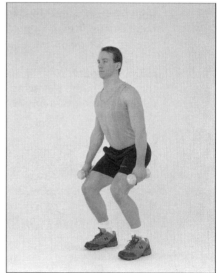

Focus & Connect: At the lowest point in the squat, focus on your butt and back thighs. To stand back up, squeeze them in unison while relaxing your shoulders, face, and hands.

Safety Tip: If your back hurts, make sure your upper body is leaning forward with a straight spine, bent at the hips (not rolling over), and bent from the lower back. If your knees hurt, make sure your hips are knee level or above and the knees are stacked above the ankles and/or mid-foot.

An outdated gym practice is to place the heels up on a raised platform while performing squats. Problem is, this encourages you to place more forward force on the knee joint — not a good thing in the long run. Because of your body positioning, you're more likely to work the thighs and get less glute work here. If you want to raise anything, let it be your toes to help push hips back. Your best bet? Keep your feet flat on the ground. Make sure your body weight is held in your heels, not your toes.

Plié Squat

The plié (see Figure 16-2), a variation of the traditional squat, is a common move used by dancers. It's also known as the 10-and-2 squat because if you were to imagine your head facing 12 o'clock on a clock, your toes would point towards 10 and 2 o'clock.

Muscles worked: Gluteals, inner thighs, quadriceps, hamstrings, erector spinae, and abs.

1. **Stand in a wide straddle position with your toes turned out to the corners. Keep your back straight and while holding weights, place your hands on your shoulders.**

   To get into the right position, pretend you're standing on an imaginary dial. Your body faces towards 12 o'clock, the right foot and right knee aim at a 2 o'clock position, the left foot and left knee aim at a 10 o'clock position.

2. **Bend your knees and lower your body, pushing your hips out slightly in back. Stop when your pelvis is at knee level. Avoid leaning into your knees.**

3. **Hold, and then contract your buttocks to straighten your legs again. Repeat.**

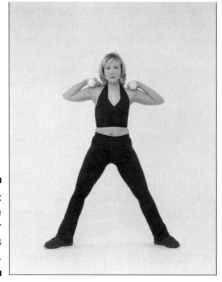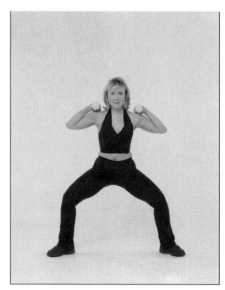

Figure 16-2:
Train like
a dancer
with this
exercise.

Focus & Connect: At the lowest point in the squat, squeeze your inner thigh muscles and your glutes to straighten back up to standing.

Safety Tip: If your knees hurt, open your legs wider and make sure that your pelvis has not sunk below knee level.

Back Lunge

You may lunge forward to go after the things you want in life, but this version of the lunge might help you pause and think before you act, because here you backtrack and take a step behind you (see Figure 16-3).

Muscles worked: Quadriceps, gluteals, hamstrings, and anterior deltoids.

1. **Stand with your feet hip-width apart and parallel. Place your hands with weights in front of your thighs, palms facing down. Hold your upper body tall.**

2. **Step back as far as you can with your left foot. Land on the back toe and avoid pushing your heel down flat to the floor.**

3. **With legs wide apart, lower your hips into a lunge position. As you lunge, raise both arms straight in front of you, stopping when they reach shoulder level.**

4. **Hold, and then push back off with the back foot to a standing position and lower your arms to your thighs. Repeat, and then switch sides.**

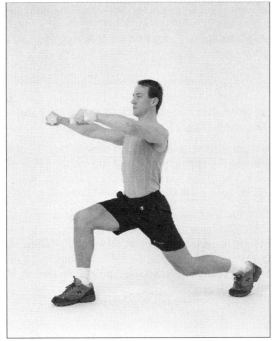

Figure 16-3:
Do enough of these butt-toning, thigh-firming moves and you might be able to reward yourself with a banana split!

Focus & Connect: At the lowest part of the lunge focus on your glutes. Contract them to return to standing.

Safety Tip: Whenever you're in the lowest position, make sure that your front knee is bent to only a 90-degree angle.

We chose the back lunge, but you can also lunge to the front. A forward lunge is as simple as taking a step forward (which we all do every day of our lives). But the deep knee bend can be problematic. This encourages you to not only step forward, but to shove all of your body weight into the front landing knee. This forward force on the knee joint is a recipe for chronic injury, so you need to be vigilant about your form. The secret to minimizing this stress is to avoid leaning your upper body forward as you lunge forward. Instead, keep your body weight distributed mostly on the back leg, as your front leg steps forward and lands lightly, heel down first.

Ab Curl

The ab curl, also called the *crunch,* may be one of the most highly performed moves of all time (and the exercise that most fitness infomercial gadgets are most likely to mimic). The key to seeing the ab firming results you want from this move is to go slower and harder, rather than faster and longer (see Figure 16-4).

Muscles worked: Rectus abdominis and transverse abdominis.

1. **Lie on your back, knees bent, feet flat. Hold your arms above your chest, palms facing each other.**

2. **Pull your bellybutton into your spine, and then move the lower part of your rib cage toward your pelvis. Bring the upper body forward, stopping when your shoulder blades are about two inches off the floor. Hold, and then lower slowly and repeat.**

   Try to perform the curl first without your hands supporting your head. However, if your neck feels strained after a few unsupported repetitions, place your hands lightly under your head. Place them wherever they are comfortable, but if they are locked behind your head, avoid pulling your head forward. Instead, rest your head back into them like a pillow.

Figure 16-4: Much of your body strength comes from developing strength at the core muscles in the abs and back.

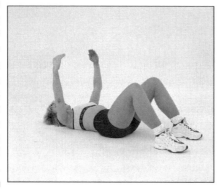 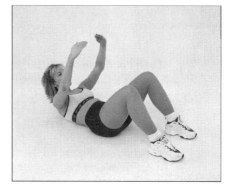

Focus & Connect: Rather than focusing on bending your spine, think of your torso as an accordion and try to scrunch up the layer of muscle down the front, decreasing the space in between your ribs and hip bones. Avoid using momentum to propel you through the moving. Move slowly feeling the muscle contraction throughout.

Safety Tip: If you suffer from lower back pain, concentrate more on flattening your abdomen than on bending your torso to raise up.

Reverse Curl

Twist your ab curl around with the reverse curl (see Figure 16-5). You'll feel like you're rocking, but try to keep this move smooth and slow.

Muscles worked: Rectus abdominis and transverse abdominis.

1. **Lie on your back with your hands by your sides. Bend your knees into your chest, and then raise your legs so that your knees are bent to a 45-degree angle — knees slightly in front of your hips and calves parallel to the floor.**

2. **Keep your head on the floor and hands by your sides, close to your body. Squeeze your bellybutton toward the floor to tilt the pelvis slightly. Hold, and then release and repeat.**

Figure 16-5:
The reverse curl shifts the emphasis to using slightly more of the muscle fibers in the lower abdominal muscles.

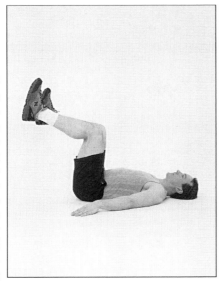 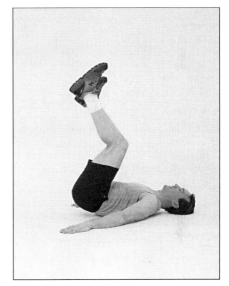

Focus & Connect: Avoid swinging the legs back and forth, instead, hold them stationary and focus on the lower ab muscles contracting fully.

Safety Tip: Avoid raising your entire lower back off the ground. Focus on the front of the torso flattening.

Push-up

If just hearing the word *push-up* makes you think boot camp, don't worry. We'll get you performing these babies faster than you can say "Hut 2-3-4!" Get on your hands and feet to try this one (see Figure 16-6).

Muscles worked: Pectorals, triceps, deltoids, and torso.

1. **Lie face down on the floor, hands just outside your shoulders, palms down, and fingers forward. Curl your feet under so your toes push against the floor.**

2. **Push your body up into a lifted prone position. Drop your hips so that your entire body is in a straight line.**

3. **Inhale and bend your elbows to lower your chest to the ground. Exhale and straighten your arms to push back up. Repeat.**

Figure 16-6:
The push-up: You're in the army now!

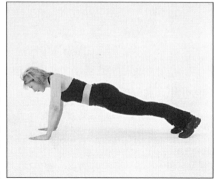 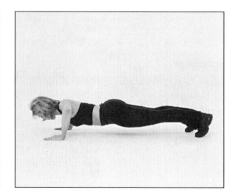

Focus & Connect: Focus on distributing your body weight equally between both feet and hands.

Options: If you're not up to supporting all of your body weight, you can train yourself to perform the push-up by gradually increasing the amount of resistance your arms push through. You can start with your hands shoulder-width apart on a window ledge or high bench. Or you can use a block to build up from supporting some of your body weight to being able to push all of it up. Start with the block just under your chest while lying on the floor. As you get stronger, move the block underneath your hips, then underneath your thighs, then calves, and then finally remove the block. By the time you've moved the block down, you should be able to complete a full body push-up easily.

Safety Tip: Avoid moving your hips up and down to simulate the push-up movement. Bend from the elbows.

Triceps Dip

Want to maximize your tube-time? Get on the sofa and do these triceps dips (see Figure 16-7) during commercial breaks. Your upper arms will get firm enough to reach for the remote and stretch for the chips with ease!

Muscles worked: Triceps and posterior deltoid.

1. **Stand in front of a bench, chair, or couch, facing away from it. Sit down on the edge and place both hands on either side of your hips, fingers forward. Supporting your body weight on your hands, raise your torso slightly and shift your body forward so that your hips are in front of the bench. Keep your feet flat and knees bent.**

2. **Bend your elbows to less than a 90-degree angle and lower your hips slightly. Hold, and then straighten the elbows to lift the body back up. Repeat.**

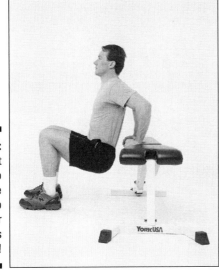 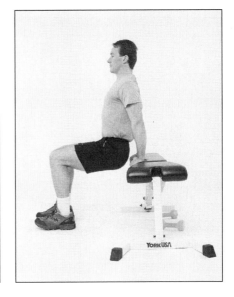

Figure 16-7: You won't need to leave the couch to keep your triceps strong!

Options: You may find it easier to balance if you straighten your legs on the floor in front of you.

Focus & Connect: Focus on the back of the upper arm, powering you through this movement.

Safety Tip: Avoid bringing the bent elbows too far behind your shoulders.

Chapter 17

Simple Muscle Moves

· ·

· ·

Some exercises are more complex than others. The pattern of each movement and position of your body determine how many muscle groups you involve during each exercise. A simple exercise, where you move one arm or leg at a time or move a part of your body in a single plane, generally means that you use fewer muscle groups. In many simple moves, the targeted muscle is said to be *isolated*. In reality, other muscles are at work helping to stabilize or assist the target muscle, but the isolated muscle is the main muscle responsible for the action of the move.

The following exercises are for the upper and lower body. We include some basic moves that we may couple together in tougher movement combinations in the following chapters. We also include a few variations to help keep the challenge in your workouts.

Lateral Raise

The lateral raise targets your shoulders. If you find that you have to arch your back to hoist the weights up, decrease to a lighter weight.

Muscles worked: Deltoids.

1. **Stand in a wide straddle position, with your feet hip-width apart. Hold weights in your hands in front of your thighs, palms facing each other.**

2. **As you exhale, contract your shoulders and raise your arms to the sides. Stop when your arms are parallel to the floor (see Figure 17-1).**

   You can also bend your knees into a plié to include some lower body action in this move (as shown in Figure 17-1).

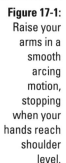

Figure 17-1:
Raise your arms in a smooth arcing motion, stopping when your hands reach shoulder level.

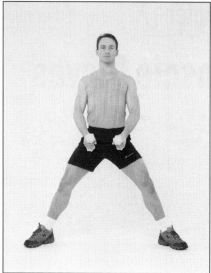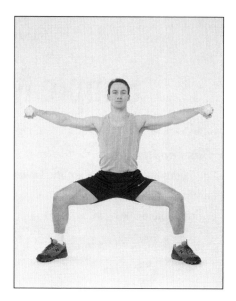

Focus & Connect: Relax your handgrip on the weights so that your hands feel light, and keep the tension in the shoulders through both the lifting and lowering phases of the move.

Safety Tip: If you find this move difficult, lift one arm at a time. If you feel excess tension in your neck, make sure to keep your shoulders down and lengthen your neck during the move. Also, keep your abdominals contracted to stabilize your torso and lead with your elbows.

Bentover Deltoid

By leaning your back slightly forward, you can raise your arms and target the back portion of your shoulder muscles. You'll also work some of your upper back with this move.

Muscles worked: Posterior deltoids and rhomboids.

1. **Stand with legs apart in a split position, both toes facing forward. Hold a weight in each hand, arms hanging in front of your body, palms facing down. First straighten your back by lifting your ribs, and then lean forward slightly from the hips. Hold your body weight back in your heels.**

2. **Exhale and open your arms out to the side, keeping the elbows bent at a 90-degree angle, lifting the weights to shoulder level. Hold, and then lower slowly and repeat. See Figure 17-2.**

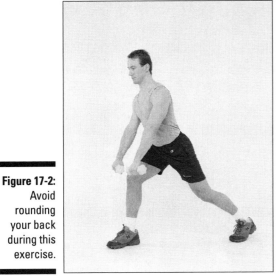 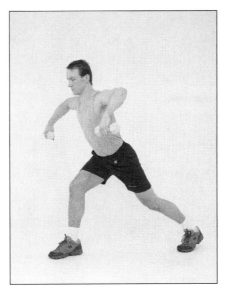

Figure 17-2:
Avoid rounding your back during this exercise.

Focus & Connect: Feel the back of your shoulder control this movement.

Safety Tip: To avoid straining your back, try not to lean too far forward; keep your chest above your waist at all times.

Military Press Overhead

By doing this move, you'll develop the strength to lift your nieces, nephews, or kids, over your head (providing they're small enough, of course!).

Muscles worked: Deltoids.

1. **Stand or sit holding weights in front of your shoulders in both hands, palms facing forward.**

2. **As you exhale, push the weights overhead, straightening the arms so that they are slightly in front of you. Hold, and then lower and repeat. See Figure 17-3.**

Focus & Connect: Before pushing the weights up, engage your shoulder blades, drawing them in together and bringing them down slightly.

Safety Tip: Try not to arch your neck by looking up; keep your chin level by looking forward.

Option: You can switch handgrips by holding the weights, palms facing forward throughout the lift.

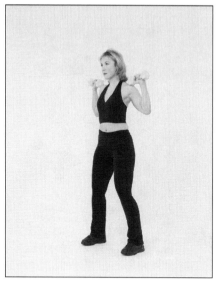 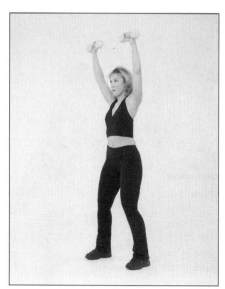

Figure 17-3:
Hold your body in perfect posture during this move by raising your rib cage and contracting your abs tight.

Triceps Kickback

Here's another great exercise to help you firm up the saggy muscle on the back of your upper arm.

Muscles worked: Triceps brachii.

1. **Stand with your feet wide apart in a split position, right in front of the left. Rest your right hand or forearm on your right thigh and lean forward with a straight back. Hold a weight in your left hand and hang it by your side. Your palm should face your body. Bend your left elbow and pull it up behind your rib cage. Hold.**

2. **Exhale and straighten your left arm behind you by straightening the elbow and moving the weight back so it stops when your arm is parallel to the floor. Keep the upper arm stable and close to your torso as you bend the elbow and lower the weight again. Repeat, and then switch arms. See Figure 17-4.**

Focus & Connect: Loosen up your handgrip so that you are holding the weight lightly; keep all the tension in the back upper arm.

Safety Tip: Avoid rounding your back as you lean forward.

Options: You can vary the handgrips in this move. In the starting position rotate your forearm inward so that your palm is facing behind you as you extend it. Then rotate your forearm outward so your palm faces forward as you extend the elbow.

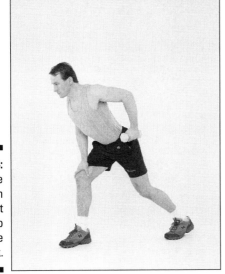 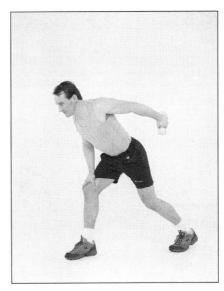

Figure 17-4:
Make sure
to rest on
the front
thigh to help
support the
lower back.

Biceps Curl

If you want to look like one of those big guys in the gym, build up your biceps
with this standard exercise for the upper arm. This is a strong muscle group
so you can probably use slightly heavier weights during this exercise.

Muscles worked: Biceps brachii, brachioradialis, and brachialis.

1. **Stand with a weight in each hand, arms hanging by your side, palms
   facing in.**

2. **Exhale, bend your elbows, and bring the weights to your shoulders.**

3. **Hold, and then slowly lower, keeping the upper arm stable and held
   close to your torso. Repeat. See Figure 17-5.**

Focus & Connect: Loosen your handgrip and focus on the powerful biceps
controlling the action.

Safety Tip: Try not to use your back to hoist the weight up. Pull your abs in
and push your weight back in your heels and hips before you lift.

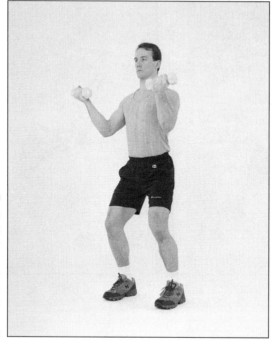

Figure 17-5:
Contract
your abs to
stabilize
your pelvis
as you curl
the weights
up.

Options:

- ✓ Change handgrips by starting with a palm facing back (forearm rotated inward) position. Then rotate the forearms outward so the palms face forward, away from your body, during the curl.

- ✓ Vary your grip. Start with your palm facing in; as you raise the weight, rotate your palm out so that it faces your shoulder at the top. During the lowering phase, rotate the palm inward to face the body. You can also start with your palm facing forward; place the side of the dumbbell against your side, and keep the palm forward throughout the motion.

- ✓ Rather than bend and straighten in the full range of motion, work through the half ranges only, first from leg to the midway point (elbow bent 90 degrees). Then work from the midway point to the closed joint position where the weight meets the shoulder.

- ✓ Complete the biceps curl with the elbow held slightly away from the body. Keep the upper arms stable and stationary throughout.

Rubber Band Row

Now's the time to use some elastic tubing or a fitness rubber band to work your back. (You can also use a dumbbell instead of a band for this move.) See Appendix B for retailers who sell these fitness products.

Muscles worked: Latissimus dorsi and posterior deltoids.

1. **Stand with your legs in a split position, right in front of left. Hold one end of a long band in each hand and loop it under your front foot so that your foot cuts the band in half. Place your arms straight by the sides of your front leg, palms facing each other. You should feel some tension in the band at this point. If you don't, wrap the slack around your hands or grab lower on the band.**

2. **Keep your back straight, abs tight, and bend your elbows to pull the band. Pull the elbows behind your rib cage and squeeze your shoulder blades together.**

3. **Hold, and then slowly lower, keeping the arms stable and held close to your torso. Repeat. See Figure 17-6.**

Focus & Connect: Rather than focusing on your hands pulling on the elastic, initiate the movement by contracting the back muscles first.

Safety Tip: Try not to bend forward at the waist, keep your back straight.

Figure 17-6:
Keep your shoulders low — not scrunched up as you pull the elbows back.

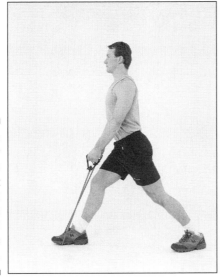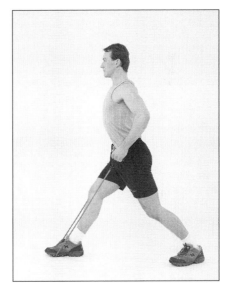

Rubber Band Back Pull

If you spend much of your day hunched over a desk, chances are your upper back muscles could use some strengthening to straighten out your posture. This exercise targets the muscles in between the shoulder blades (see Figure 17-7).

Muscles worked: Rhomboids.

1. **Stand with your legs in a straddle position. Hold one end of a long band in each hand, then bunch up the ends and hold it close to the center of the band so that when you extend your arms straight in front of you, shoulder-width apart; there is no slack. You should feel some tension in the band at this point. If you don't, grab lower on the band.**

2. **Keep your back straight, abs tight, and pull the band out to each side by opening your arms wider.**

3. **Squeeze your shoulder blades together. Hold, and then repeat.**

Focus & Connect: Keep your shoulders low as your contract the upper back muscles.

Safety Tip: Maintain perfect posture. Draw your shoulder blades together, and lower them down by dropping your shoulders.

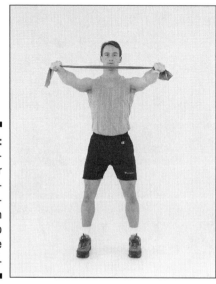 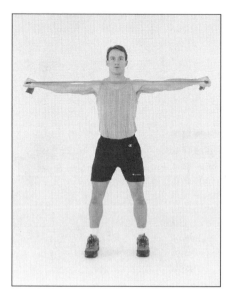

Figure 17-7: In this exercise, your back muscles contract in order to stretch the band.

Static Single Leg Extension

Unless you're a dancer or a gymnast, doing exercises to improve your balance is often the one thing people leave out of their exercise training. However, it's vital for total body control, especially during sports where you are twisting, turning, and shifting your body weight all over the place. This exercise should be held for as long as possible with perfect posture (see Figure 17-8).

Muscles worked: Hip flexors, quadriceps, and gluteals.

1. **Stand with both feet hip-width apart and hands holding weights by your sides. Raise your right leg in front. Keep it straight and lift slowly up as high as you can without tilting your pelvis or losing balance. Hold. Then, very slowly lower down, keeping your hips and torso stable throughout.**

2. **Perform the same movement, but this time when your leg reaches the high point, steady your body and rotate your thigh outward. Hold, and then rotate the thigh inward and lower slowly (not shown). Repeat, and then switch legs.**

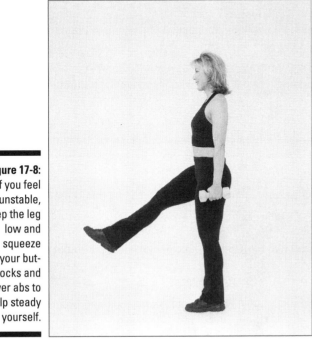

Figure 17-8:
If you feel unstable, keep the leg low and squeeze your buttocks and lower abs to help steady yourself.

Focus & Connect: Spread the toes out for a stable base of support in your standing leg, and then relax the foot of your extended leg and initiate all the action from the quads.

Safety Tip: Avoid letting your upper body slump; hold your ribs high and lengthen your spine throughout.

Standing Side Leg Lift

Here's another balancing move where your weight shifts sideways. You'll know that your ab and back muscles are strong if you can perform balancing moves without wobbling.

Muscles worked: Gluteals and hip abductors.

1. **Stand with your feet hip-width apart, toes forward, hands by your sides.**

2. **Raise your left hand to your chest, bending and raising your left arm so that your elbow points out sideways, stopping at shoulder level. At the same time, open your right arm straight to the side until it's parallel to the floor. Open your right leg out to the side and raise it 45 degrees off the floor. Avoid tilting your pelvis. Keep the knee facing forward. Hold, and then slowly lower and repeat. Switch legs. See Figure 17-9.**

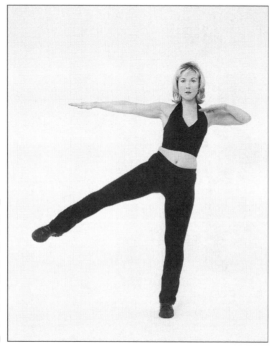

Figure 17-9:
Tighten your abs and buttocks to prevent throwing your torso off-kilter.

Focus & Connect: Balance throughout this move by lengthening your spine and squeezing your glutes.

Safety Tip: Relax your shoulders and avoid holding your breath.

Option: While balanced on one leg, bend your supporting leg into a semi-squat to lower your hips slightly. Hold, and then straighten the leg.

Ab Crunch on Ball

Here's a great way to take your ab exercises to the next level. Your gym will probably have stability balls, which are large rubber balls. If not, you can buy one from your local sporting goods store or from one of the retailers listed in Appendix B.

Muscles worked: Rectus abdominis.

1. **Sit on top of a stability ball. Lie back and position yourself so that you balance your mid-to-low back on the top of the ball. With knees bent and feet flat, walk your feet away from the ball so that your knees form a 90-degree angle and your thighs are parallel to the floor. Aim your arms straight to the ceiling, or if that's too difficult, rest your hands behind your head. Drop your head and upper body back so that you're extended along the slope of the ball.**

2. **As you exhale, contract your abs by pulling your bellybutton in and move your rib cage toward your hips to curl forward.**

3. **Hold, and then slowly lower into the outstretched position and repeat. See Figure 17-10.**

Focus & Connect: Feel all the muscles in your torso interact to keep your body stable.

Safety Tip: If you feel unstable, move your body along the ball so that your hips and low back are over the downward slope of the ball.

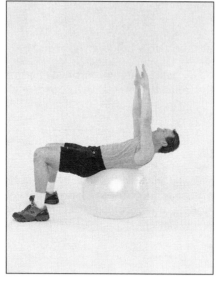 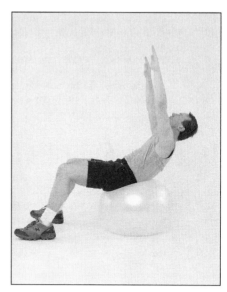

Figure 17-10:
The ball will wobble a bit, causing your muscles to work harder to stabilize you.

Ab Twist on Ball

This move adds a challenging twist to the ab crunch on the ball. Remember not to pull on your head but to focus on rotating your torso instead.

Muscles worked: Rectus abdominis.

1. **Sit on top of a stability ball. Lie back and position yourself so that you balance your mid-to-low back on the top of the ball. Walk your feet away from the ball so that your thighs are parallel to the floor. Reach your hands straight above your head. If that's too difficult, place your hands behind or on the sides of your head. Drop your head and upper body back and pull your rib cage away from your pelvis.**

2. **As you exhale, pull your bellybutton in and curl forward. Then twist your rib cage to the right. Hold, and then slowly lower into the out-stretched position, curl forward, and twist to the left. Keep your hips stationary as your upper body turns. Repeat. See Figure 17-11.**

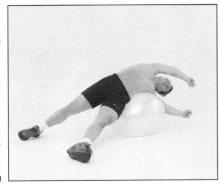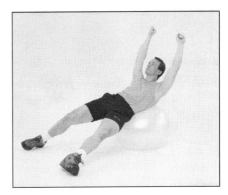

Figure 17-11:
Stretch all
the way
back on the
ball before
raising and
rotating your
upper body.

Focus & Connect: Feel the lower abdominals contract to maintain torso balance as you lift, turn, and lower.

Safety Tip: Avoid turning your neck or pulling on your head if your hands are supporting it.

Back Extension

This exercise targets the lower back and buttocks. It can be done on the floor, but you'll get a better range of motion if you hang off a bench.

Muscles worked: Erector spinae and gluteals.

1. **Lie face down with your legs straddling a bench, or if you are on the floor, place your legs straight and stretch your arms along the floor over your head. On the bench, scoot your upper body off the top end so that as much of your upper half is hanging off the side as is comfortable. Place your hands behind your head.**

2. **As you exhale, squeeze your buttocks and raise your upper body (including your arms) to 3-6 inches above the horizontal line where your back is parallel to the floor. Hold, and then lower and repeat. See Figure 17-12.**

Figure 17-12:
Move slowly
during both
the lifting
and lower-
ing phases
of this move.

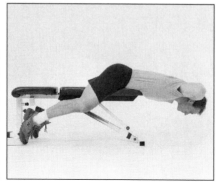 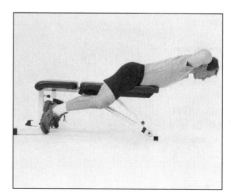

Focus & Connect: Relax your hands, feet, and shoulders. Feel the back muscles getting stronger throughout the movement.

Safety Tip: Look down, not forward, to avoid arching your neck. If you feel any discomfort in your lower back, raise only your arms. Keep your back and head down and your forehead to the floor.

Chapter 18

Multimuscle Moves

· ·

In This Chapter

▶ Challenging whole-body moves

▶ Functional exercises

· ·

*I*n this chapter, you can take the basic movements to the next level by adding more resistance and more whole-body movement to the exercises. These moves tend to be more functional, mimicking actions you might perform in sports or even in everyday life.

Walking Lunge

The walking lunge is a standard lower body strength exercise that helps you improve your balance. Watch your form during this move because it's easy to push too much body weight into your knee as you step to the front.

Muscles worked: Quadriceps, hamstrings, and gluteals.

1. **Start with your feet hip-width apart and parallel.**

2. **Step your right foot forward as far as you can.**

3. **As your heel lands, lower your hips into a lunge position.**

   Keep the front knee bent at no less than 90 degrees.

4. **Squeeze the glutes and hamstrings of the front leg to bring your back leg forward to a standing position. Then step forward with the left leg.**

Focus & Connect: Land lightly with each forward step — feel like a feather.

Safety Tip: Hold your body weight in your back foot as you take each forward step to avoid straining the front knee.

Walk-Thru Lunge

The walk-thru lunge takes the basic walking lunge one step further by eliminating the pausing phase in between steps. Lunge like you're walking, alternating feet with each step.

Muscles worked: Quadriceps, hamstrings, and gluteals.

1. **Start with your feet hip-width apart and parallel, hands on your hips.**

2. **Step your right foot forward as far as you can.**

3. **As your heel lands, lower your hips into a lunge position. See Figure 18-1.**

   Keep the front knee bent at no less than 90 degrees.

4. **Now bring the back leg forward to immediately step forward into a left lunge.**

Focus & Connect: At the deepest part of each step, imagine that you're knee-deep in mud; ignite the powerful action of your front glutes and quads to take the next step.

Safety Tip: Avoid excess stress on the front knee by making each forward step as wide as possible.

Figure 18-1:
The walk-thru lunge is similar to the walking lunge.

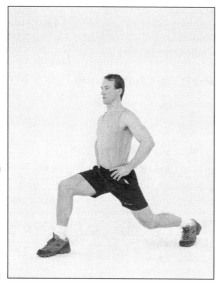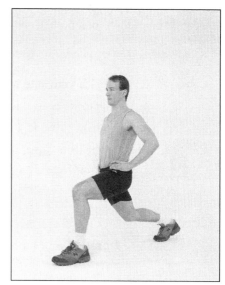

Weighted Walking Lunge

If you've been going through the last two exercises in order, you're probably noticing a pattern, right? If you're starting to think that the last two moves were cake walks, get ready for this one! The weighted walking lunge adds more resistance and some upper body movement that forces your torso to work even harder to stay stabilized.

Muscles worked: Quadriceps, hamstrings, gluteals, deltoids, and latissimus dorsi.

1. **Start with your feet hip-width apart and parallel. Hold a light weight (about 3-8 pounds) with both hands on the right side of your body near your thigh. See Figure 18-2.**

2. **Step your left foot forward as far in front as you can. At the same time, lift the weight up in front to about waist level and cross it over the front of your body to bring it to the outside of your bent knee.**

3. **As your heel lands, lower your hips into a lunge position.**

   Keep the front knee bent at no less than 90 degrees.

4. **Now bring the back leg forward to immediately step forward into a right lunge, shifting the weight back to the other side.**

Focus & Connect: Feel your arm, front thigh, and body rise and lower together.

Safety Tip: Keep the focus on front knee alignment once your arm starts moving.

Figure 18-2: Move slowly as you lunge to control the placement of your front knee and to balance your moving body.

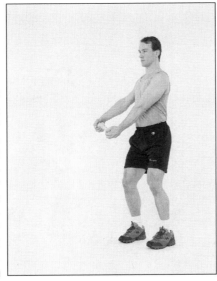
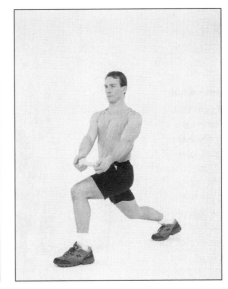

Side Lunge

Many sports require that you shift your weight side to side. The side lunge helps prepare you for it, but watch your form so that you don't stress your knees.

Muscles worked: Abductors, adductors, quadriceps, hamstrings, and anterior deltoids.

1. **Stand with your feet wider than hip-width, toes pointing forward.**

2. **Lower your body into a squat position by pushing your hips back. See Figure 18-3.**

   Hands should hang straight in front of your thighs with your palms down.

3. **Leading with your left heel, lift your left thigh and move your leg to the left, taking a step to the side. Land on your heel gently.**

4. **Lower your arms as you lift your body and bring your right foot to the left.**

5. **Repeat, and then switch directions.**

Focus & Connect: Keep your body balanced with your weight in your heels as you lift and lower.

Safety Tip: Be aware of the knee you land on; push your hips back at all times to avoid increasing the pressure in your knee.

Options: Hold weights during the arm movements.

Figure 18-3:
Step carefully to the side, keeping your body weight in the heels, so that you don't put too much pressure on your knees.

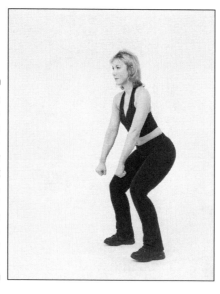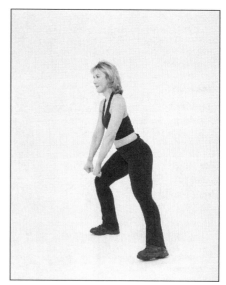

Dynamic Side Lunge

The dynamic side lunge takes the basic side lunge a step further by adding a hop to the sideways movement. Keep the jump low and your feet close together.

Muscles worked: Hip abductors, hip adductors, quadriceps, and hamstrings.

1. **Stand with your feet hip-width, toes pointing forward.**

2. **Lower your body into a squat position by pushing your hips back, and hold your hands behind your head. Shift your body weight over to your left foot and lift the right heel up so your right toes an help you balance. See Figure 18-4.**

3. **Leading with your right foot, hop and shift your body to the right, lifting your right thigh and moving your leg to the right (see the right photo in Figure 18-4). Land on your heel gently and keep the weight in your right foot.**

4. **Repeat the hops from side to side.**

Focus & Connect: Keep the lower body movement smooth.

Figure 18-4:
Focus on keeping your movement under control as you shift your weight from side to side.

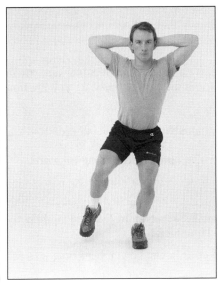 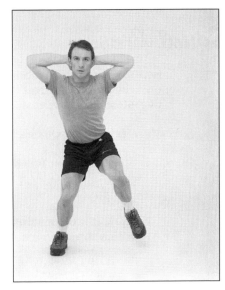

Back Lunge with Forward Raise

Lunging backwards is a good alternative to doing them forward. You'll be less likely to push your knees too far forward.

Muscles worked: Gluteals, quadriceps, hamstrings, and deltoids.

1. **Stand with your feet shoulder-width apart, feet parallel.**

   Your hands should be holding weights straight in front of your thighs, palms down.

2. **Step back with your right leg and lower your body into a back lunge. At the same time, raise the arms in front to shoulder level.**

3. **Squeeze the front glutes to bring your back leg forward.**

4. **Step back with the other leg. Repeat.**

Focus & Connect: Hold your back upright or lean slightly forward as you step back, landing only on the back toe, not the heel.

Safety Tip: Step back far enough so the front knee bends only to a 90-degree angle.

Squat Press

Here's a move that combines two basic moves, the squat and the military press overhead, to target the upper and lower body. As you sit, imagine sitting into an invisible chair.

Muscles worked: Quadriceps, hamstrings, gluteals, and deltoids.

1. **Start with your feet hip-width apart, toes facing forward.**

   Hold your hands with weights near your shoulders, palms facing each other.

2. **Squat low by pushing your hips back and leaning slightly forward with a straight back. See Figure 18-5.**

   Keep your body weight in your heels. Lower your buttocks as if you were sitting in a chair.

3. **Squeeze your glutes and raise your body to the standing position. At the same time, push the weights overhead to straighten your arms.**

4. **Lower back into the squat and repeat.**

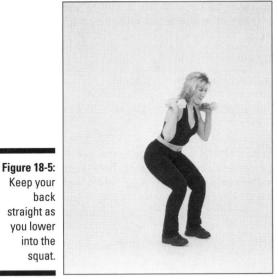

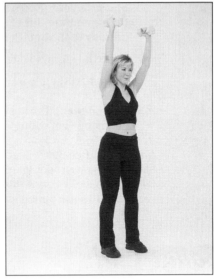

Figure 18-5:
Keep your
back
straight as
you lower
into the
squat.

Focus & Connect: Lengthen your spine as you stand up and extend your arms.

Safety Tip: Keep the knees over the ankles, not toes, at the deepest point in the squat.

Plié with Arm Raise

A *plié* is the French word for this position in which you stand in a wide squat with your toes turned out. We combine the lower body move with a shoulder exercise.

Muscles worked: Quadriceps, hamstrings, gluteals, and deltoids.

1. **Start with your feet wider than hip-width apart, toes facing out to the corners.**

   Hold your hands with weights in front of your thighs, palms facing each other.

2. **Squat low by pushing your hips back and leaning slightly forward with a straight back.**

   Keep your body weight in your heels, and rotate your thighs and feet outward slightly so that your knees aim to the corners, rather than straight ahead of your body.

3. **Squeeze your glutes and raise your body to the standing position. At the same time, lift the weights out to the sides, stopping when your hands reach shoulder level.**

   Keep the elbows soft, palms forward or down.

4. **Hold, and then lower arms and body slowly. Repeat.**

Focus & Connect: During the lifting phase, squeeze the shoulders and glutes while relaxing everything else.

Safety Tip: Because added arm movement may distract you, maintain constant focus on proper knee alignment during knee bends: bend your knees at 90 degrees, hold your weight in the heels, and keep your calves almost perpendicular to the floor.

Squat Curls

Flex your arms as you sit low, and then squeeze your buttocks tight to stand up with perfect posture as you perform this squat curl.

Muscles worked: Biceps brachii, quadriceps, hamstrings, and gluteals.

1. **Start with your feet hip-width apart, toes facing forward. See Figure 18-6.**

   Hold your weights near the outside of your thighs, palms facing forward.

2. **Squat low by pushing your hips back and leaning slightly forward with a straight back. At the same time, lift the weights by bending the elbows into a biceps curl. Bring the elbows slightly in front of your torso.**

   Keep your body weight in your heels.

3. **Squeeze your glutes and raise your body to the standing position as you straighten your elbows, lowering the weights by your sides.**

4. **Repeat.**

Focus & Connect: Keep your body weight in your heels and squeeze the buttocks throughout.

Safety Tip: As you stand, avoid arching your back to hoist the hand weights up.

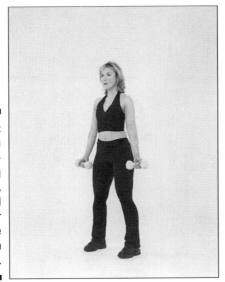 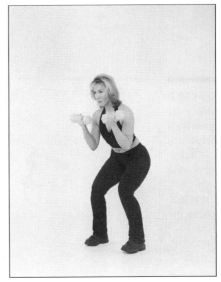

Figure 18-6:
When you lean forward during the squat, don't round your back or bend at the waist. Lean from the hip.

Options:

> ✔ Start with the hands in a hammer grip with your palms facing in throughout the move.

> ✔ Start with the hands turning inwards with your palms facing behind you.

Lunge Scissor Kick

The lunge scissor kick looks like a difficult move, but once you've got the hang of it, it's really quite easy.

Muscles worked: Quadriceps, gluteals, and hamstrings.

1. **Stand with your feet together, hip-width apart.**

2. **Lunge your right leg back. At the same time, bring your right arm up in front and left arm straight by your side to the back. See Figure 18-7.**

3. **As you squeeze your left glutes and hamstrings to straighten, raise your right leg up in front of your body and kick forward to hip level or below as your right arm swings back and left arm swings front.**

4. **Hold, and then lower slowly.**

5. **Repeat, and then switch sides.**

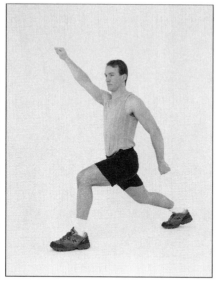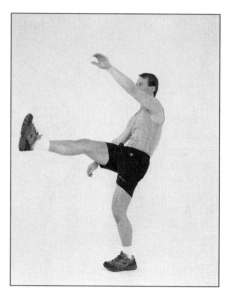

Figure 18-7:
Kick below knee level until you are flexible enough in your hamstrings to increase the range of motion to hip level.

Focus & Connect: Feel the opposite side of your body move in unison.

Safety Tip: Make sure that you keep your kick low and controlled, especially if your hamstrings are tight.

Chop Squat

The chop squat incorporates upper and lower body movement with a little twist that will activate your abdominal muscles to help stabilize your body.

Muscles worked: Quadriceps, gluteals, hamstrings, and deltoids.

1. **Stand with your feet hip-width apart, toes pointing forward.**

2. **Lower your body into a squat position by pushing your hips back. Hold weights in both hands by the left thigh. See Figure 18-8.**

3. **Keeping the abs tight, straighten your legs to stand, and kick your left leg out to the side as you raise your arms from the lower left toward the upper-right corner.**

4. **Lower your arms and leg to the squat again.**

5. **Repeat, and then switch sides.**

Focus & Connect: Maintain body equilibrium as your arms and leg move to opposite sides.

Safety Tip: Push your hips slightly back every time you bend your knees.

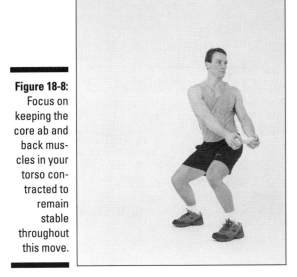 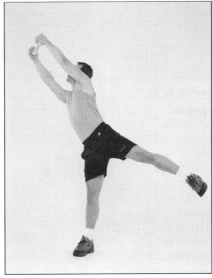

Figure 18-8:
Focus on keeping the core ab and back muscles in your torso contracted to remain stable throughout this move.

One Leg Squat Press

The one leg squat press requires some strength, coordination, and control. You'll shift your weight from side to side and raise one leg to the side. Move slowly so that you can execute this one with precise technique.

Muscles worked: Deltoids, gluteals, quadriceps, and hamstrings.

1. **Stand with your feet hip-width apart, toes pointing forward.**

2. **Lower your body into a side lunge position by pushing your hips toward the right and holding your body weight in your right leg. Hold weights in both hands above your shoulders and out to the sides. See Figure 18-9.**

   Your elbows should be bent so that your arms form a rectangle.

3. **As you exhale, push your body weight into your left foot to stand and open your right leg out to the side as you push both arms overhead.**

4. **Lower your arms and leg.**

5. **Repeat, and then switch sides.**

Focus & Connect: Activate your back muscles to keep your spine erect and limbs extended during the upward phase.

Safety Tip: When you lower, hold your back up high, rather than leaning over into a flat back.

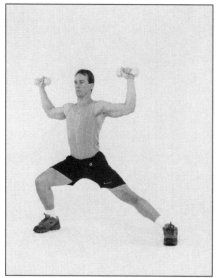 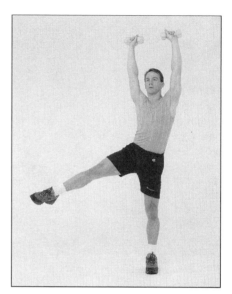

Figure 18-9: Hold this position at the top for five seconds when you're out-stretched to improve your ability to balance.

Standing Good Morning

The good morning move is great for targeting your buttocks to straighten your body back up to a standing position; however, you may feel strain on your back. If you do, limit how far you bend forward and keep your knees slightly bent.

Muscles worked: Erector spinae and gluteals.

1. **Stand tall with your feet shoulder-width apart. Hold weights in your hands on the outside of your thighs, palms down. See Figure 18-10.**

2. **Squeeze your glutes and lower abs.**

3. **Inhale and press your chest out in front to lean forward with a straight back. Stop when your torso reaches between 45 to 90 degrees of flexion.**

4. **Contract the glutes to straighten up.**

5. **Repeat slowly.**

Focus & Connect: Lengthen your spine as you lean forward.

Safety Tip: If your back hurts, bend your knees and lean only to 45 degrees or less.

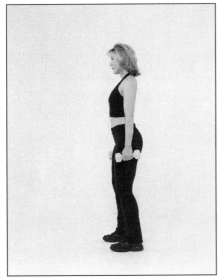 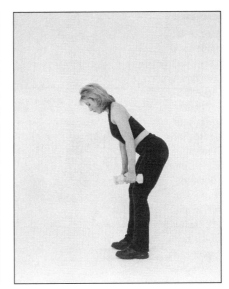

Figure 18-10:
When you lean forward, contract the abs by pulling your bellybutton in to help support your lower back.

Lower Body Ball Twist

The *stability ball,* also known as the Swiss ball, is a great tool for doing ab work. This move causes your core abdominal muscles to contract in order to move the ball.

Muscles worked: Rectus abdominis and obliques.

1. **Lie on your back with your knees bent and feet flat. Hold a stability ball (any size) in between your legs. Open your arms out to the sides with your palms flat on the floor. See Figure 18-11.**

2. **Exhale as you pull your bellybutton in and lower your legs to the right. Stabilize your body by pressing your upper arms into the floor.**

3. **Hold, and then contract the abs to bring the thighs in again.**

4. **Lower to the other side. Then repeat.**

Focus & Connect: Keep the upper body still and relaxed as you tense the lower abs.

Safety Tip: To avoid back strain, keep your movement slow and your knees close to your body.

Figure 18-11:
If your back
is tight, you
may find it
uncomfort-
able to
lower your
legs too far
to either
side.
Decrease
the range of
motion and
focus on
squeezing
your abs
tight.

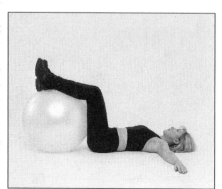
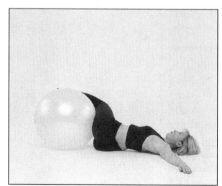

Chapter 19

Key Gym Equipment

. . . .

In This Chapter

▶ The essential gym machines you should use

▶ Free weight exercises you can do on a bench

. . . .

*W*hen you walk into a gym, the array of shiny exercise machines can dazzle you with their training potential — or overwhelm you with confusion. With exercise, variety is key, and you can choose from hundreds of different moves. Since your muscles always benefit from adding surprise challenges, doing similar moves in different ways with different equipment is always a good idea. This book includes the moves that we've found to be most effective, but that in no way means that you won't benefit by trying lots of different variations of exercises.

For the most part, we've stuck to *free weight* exercises using dumbbells. Not only can you do these at home if you don't have access to a health club, free weights also are generally a better way to train because your body gets a workout stabilizing itself during each exercise. In most cases, you can target the same muscle groups with a pair of dumbbells that you can with resistance machines in the gym. However, a few exercises can't be replicated very easily with free weights, such as the lat pulldown or cable pulley moves, so you need special gym equipment to perform those.

We picked the gym moves we like best, both on resistance machines and using free weights on a bench. But remember, most bench moves can also be performed on the type of step used in step aerobics classes. Sometimes you can do a similar move on a table, chair, or your bed at home, but you need to make sure that whatever you use is extremely sturdy and supportive.

When you use a gym machine, the amount of weight you lift will be different from the amount you might use when holding dumbbells. You'll probably have to redetermine your starting weights for each new machine you try. Review Chapter 14 for guidelines on how much weight to use. In general, you want to make sure that by the end of 8-12 repetitions your target muscles feel fatigued. If you can do more than 15 repetitions of an exercise, you're training for endurance, not strength; you may wish to work with heavier weights to challenge the muscles.

Using Resistance Machines

Resistance machines come in many shapes, styles, and sizes. In some cases, several machines work the same muscle groups and perform the same basic exercises, but they put you in different positions (sitting, lying, or standing), so the machines may look different. Some equipment uses a series of cables to pull up different amounts of weight bars stacked on top of each other. Other equipment uses hydraulic resistance — air pressure — to provide the resistance that your muscles will move against. A few machines, such as the Pilates Reformer, use springs for resistance. Whatever the physics of the machine you use, they all operate on the same principle: They make your muscles produce extra force to overcome the resistance. Weight machines are the best type to allow you to monitor your progression — you can be very specific when determining the amount of weight and the increases in overload that you choose.

Lat pulldown

Since most free weight exercises with dumbbells have you raise the weight up, this machine is useful because the resistance is in the opposite direction. You pull away from the resistance instead of bringing it toward you.

Muscles worked: Latissimus dorsi.

1. **Choose your desired weight, and then grasp the handles of the pull-down bar and sit on the seat of the machine. Extend your arms fully in a V position. Face your palms forward, not up, and curl your thumbs around the bar.**

2. **Sit and lean back slightly, and then exhale and pull the bar down, lowering it to the front of your chest with your elbows pressed to your sides. You may need to lean your torso slightly back, but keep the spine straight and abdominals contracted. Keep your wrists straight, in line with your forearms.**

3. **Hold, and then inhale as you allow the bar to raise up slowly. Repeat.**

Focus & Connect: Rather than concentrating on your hands pulling on the bar, think of squeezing your back and shoulder muscles first to move the bar.

Safety Tip: Although you'll still see people in the gym using this machine incorrectly, avoid pulling the bar behind your neck as the position puts extreme stress on the shoulder joint.

Cable row

This is another pulling exercise that is great for the entire back. Make sure to hold good posture throughout: Keep your ribs lifted and spine straight.

Muscles worked: Latissimus dorsi, rhomboids, and posterior deltoids.

1. **Choose your desired weight, and then attach the appropriate bar. The cable machine has several differently shaped handles that allow you to move in different directions, and with one or two hands.**

2. **Hold onto one bar with each hand and stand facing the weight stack. Your legs are in a split stance, right leg in front of the left. Your arms should extend in front of you at thigh level with your palms facing in.**

3. **As you exhale, pull your elbows toward your rib cage, and then behind your back. Hold, and then return to the extended position and repeat.**

Focus & Connect: Feel your shoulder blades come together as your arms pull back.

Safety Tip: Avoid slouching, hold your ribs lifted, and keep your spine straight.

Cable press

This pulling exercise targets your chest muscles.

Muscles worked: Pectorals, deltoids, and serratus anterior.

1. **Select your desired weight and stand sideways, left side next to a cable machine. Hold onto the cable handle with your inside (left) hand. Walk away from the machine until your left arm is outstretched; keep your elbow soft. Let your palm face down. Soften your knees, and with a straight back, lean slightly forward.**

2. **As you exhale, pull on the cable to move your arm across the front of your body, stopping when your left hand reaches the right side of your body. Hold, and then move the arm to the left side again and repeat.**

3. **Switch sides.**

Focus & Connect: Feel the chest area near the inner upper arm contract as you move the weight.

Safety Tip: Avoid rounding your upper back. Keep the spine straight and abs tight throughout.

Pull-up bar

At it's simplest, a pull-up bar is just a stable horizontal bar above your head that you reach up and grab onto to pull your head above the bar (similar to the bars you'll find on the jungle gym at the playground). This is a very difficult exercise because you essentially have to raise all of your body weight up, which can be a lot if you haven't worked up to it. Some new assisted pull-up machines in the gym allow you to lift up a portion of your weight. This enables you to work up gradually to doing full unassisted pull-ups. You can also make the standard pull-up easier by placing a chair underneath so that you pull yourself up from a higher level to begin with.

Muscles worked: Trapezius, latissimus dorsi, biceps, and deltoids.

1. **Stand just underneath, but slightly behind an overhead bar. Hold onto the bar with your hands spaced shoulder-width apart. Your palms should face forward, and your thumbs should curl under.**

2. **As you exhale, pull your body up so that your chin rises above the bar by bending your elbows and using your back muscles to draw the elbows close to your ribs. Hold, and then slowly lower and repeat.**

Options: To target different areas of the muscle groups, switch grips. Try a wider grip, hands spaced about three inches away from each shoulder. Or try a reverse grip with the palms rotated inward so that they face your body when grasping the bar.

Focus & Connect: Tighten your abs and entire torso to keep your body stable throughout the lift.

Safety Tip: If this is too difficult at first, start from the top and work your way down. Step up onto a bench, hold yourself in a lifted position, and then lower down slowly. When you can successfully lower with control, remove the bench and go through both the lifting and lowering phases of the move. You can also try the assisted pull-up machines in the gym that allow you to adjust how much of your own body weight you lift during the exercise.

Triceps cable extension

You can work your triceps in a multitude of positions using free weights. Here's a variation on the cable machine.

Muscles worked: Triceps brachii and posterior deltoids.

1. **Choose your desired weight, and stand in front of the cable machine. Grasp onto the bar with both hands (palms down) and lower it so that it is in front of your waist. Your elbows should be bent at 90 degrees, and fists should be in front of your elbows.**

2. **As you exhale, push your hands down so that your elbows straighten. Keep your elbows by your sides and upper arm stable throughout the move. Hold, and then slowly raise the weight to starting position and repeat.**

Focus & Connect: Tighten your abs and stand up tall (ribs lifted, thighs straight) during the move.

Safety Tip: If your elbows feel strained, make sure your hands are spaced elbow-width apart on the bar and/or lighten your weight.

Warming the Bench

The incline bench is a versatile piece of equipment that allows you to change the angles of your body. We like the fact that you can adjust how you sit or lie because it helps you target different (and more) muscle fibers. In many cases, you can do these same exercises on an aerobic step at home.

Incline chest press

Remember the Right Angle Rule when getting into position for the incline chest press.

Muscles worked: Pectorals and deltoids.

1. **Adjust the bench to your desired level of incline (experiment with 15 to 45 degrees). Sit on the bench and hold weights in each hand. Bend your elbows to 90 degrees. Keep your upper arms at shoulder level, your palms facing forward, and your wrists straight. See Figure 19-1.**

   As you exhale, push the weights directly up to extend your arms. Keep palms facing forward. Hold, and then bend elbows and lower weights to the side again. Repeat.

Focus & Connect: Squeeze your upper inner arms as if you were hugging a giant beach ball.

Safety Tip: Avoid arching your lower back or locking your elbows as you raise the weight.

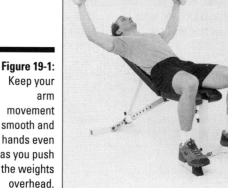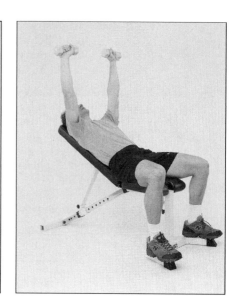

Figure 19-1:
Keep your arm movement smooth and hands even as you push the weights overhead.

Triceps press

This positions targets a large portion of your triceps, compared to the other triceps exercises.

Muscles worked: Triceps brachii.

1. **Lie on your back on a bench. The bench can be horizontal or placed on an incline. Bend your knees and place your feet flat on the bench or floor. Hold one dumbbell in each hand, or if you prefer a lighter weight, one dumbbell in both hands. Straighten your arms and raise them over your head so that the arms form a straight line pointing above or slightly behind your head. See Figure 19-2.**

2. **Bend your elbows and drop your hands behind your shoulders. Exhale and straighten your arms, keeping them in a diagonal line.**

3. **Bend and repeat.**

Focus & Connect: Keep your upper arms stable throughout and focus on tightening the back of the upper arm when your arms are straight.

Safety Tip: If your elbows feel strained, lighten your weight.

Options: You may also do this exercise one arm at a time, lying or sitting on the bench.

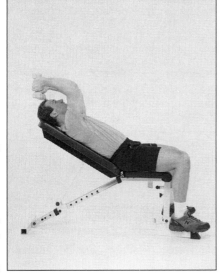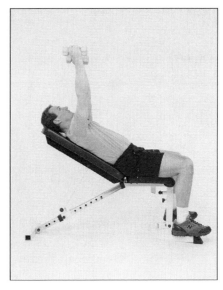

Figure 19-2:
Tighten the back of the upper arm as your elbow straightens.

Reverse back extension

If you have a healthy back, this exercise can help strengthen your lower back muscles. Perform it slowly, and stop if you feel any strain in the spine.

Muscles worked: Gluteals and erector spinae.

1. **Lie face down on a flat bench and turn your head to one side. Your hips should lie on the edge of the lower end of the bench. Hang your legs off the end of the bench. Your thighs should be at a 90-degree angle to your hips. Bend the knees. Grab onto the supporting legs or front ledge of the bench with your arms, or wrap your hands around the bench in a bear hug for support. See Figure 19-3.**

2. **As you exhale, squeeze your buttocks and slowly raise both legs up until they are horizontal. Hold, and then slowly lower and repeat.**

Focus & Connect: Think of your feet to back as one unit during the lift.

Safety Tip: If this is too difficult, shift your body higher along the bench so that you lift less of your legs.

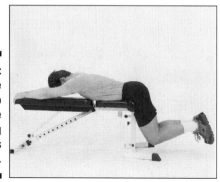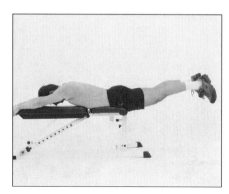

Figure 19-3:
Tighten the buttocks to raise the legs during this exercise.

Inclined bentover row

The inclined bentover row works your upper back. Really concentrate on bringing your shoulder blades together to make the most of this move.

Muscles worked: Deltoids and rhomboids.

1. **Lie face down on an inclined bench. Holding a weight in each hand, hang your arms down off the sides of the bench, palms facing in. (See Figure 19-4.)**

2. **As you exhale, pull your elbows into your waist and behind your body. Inhale as you slowly lower. Repeat.**

Focus & Connect: Imagine your shoulder blades coming together as your elbows point up.

Safety Tip: Keep your chin low to avoid arching your neck.

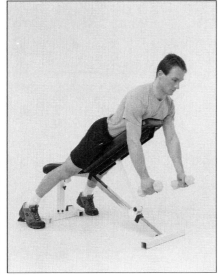 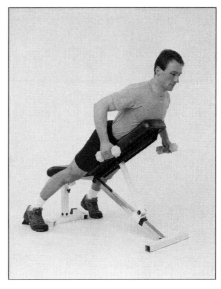

Figure 19-4:
Squeeze the back muscles during this exercise.

Chapter 20

Power Moves

In This Chapter

▶ Explosive moves to get you superfit

▶ Dynamic training (high energy, explosive, and fast)

*I*n our everyday lives, most of us are pretty lazy. On occasion though, we have to sprint wildly to catch the bus or catch our balance to prevent a precarious slip on a wet floor. If we play sports — whether it's tennis or football — the ability to make quick turns, dashes, stops, and starts is all part of the game. The physical prowess that this type of fitness entails is quick reflex actions and the ability to move fast in a second's notice (and then stop your sudden acceleration just as quickly). Since fitness is specific (Part II explains why), your long slow walks aren't going to cut it when it comes to developing your fitness level in this area. Instead of waiting until you're leaping to catch a touchdown pass before you decide to practice, we help prepare you by including some dynamic ways to train in this and the next chapter. These are movements that require high amounts of quick energy either from moving really fast or from adding small jumps.

As well as some faster strength moves, we add a couple of plyometric — or explosive jumping — exercises that you can do in a controlled environment. But only the fittest and the most athletic should try them. Because they are so explosive, plyometric moves are challenging — and risky. You should never (and, we repeat, never) try these drills if you have any sort of orthopedic or joint injuries that may be worsened by the stress of the impact. And if you're a beginner, you should get in shape first before you attempt to do them. You won't have the necessary muscle control, strength, and balance to execute these moves properly. So any gains you get from doing them may be outweighed by the stress of overuse on your joints. In the next chapter, we include more high energy moves: sprint and coordination drills.

You should do fewer repetitions of these moves than you would normally do during strength exercises. Some athletes have been known to use weights when performing these moves, but unless you have your own personal strength coach, personal trainer, or physical therapist watching over you, we wouldn't recommend it for general exercisers.

If, during any of these moves, your knees, ankles, feet, or back hurt, the exercise is not for you. If you are overweight or are a man who weighs more than 200 pounds, you shouldn't do any plyometric exercises.

Jump Lunge

When you were a kid, you probably played leapfrog, hopped around like a rabbit, or sprung up on other unsuspecting kids while playing hide-and-seek. This move (see Figure 20-1) takes a basic lunge and adds a fun jump to it.

Muscles worked: Gluteals, quadriceps, hamstrings, abdominals, and calves.

1. **Stand with your feet in a split position: right leg in front of your body, left leg in back, and torso positioned evenly in the middle of the two. Both toes should be pointing forward. Hold your hands behind your head, and keep your elbows opened out to the sides.**

2. **Lower your body slightly by bending the knees and dropping your hips.**

3. **With a spurt of power, use your thighs to spring up vertically in the air and scissor your legs midway. Land with the opposite leg in front.**

Focus & Connect: Hold your rib cage high, and contract the abs as you feel your glutes power you through this move.

Safety Tip: Try to minimize the impact of landing by keeping your knees soft, distributing your body weight from heel to toe and landing softly.

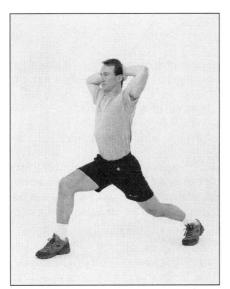 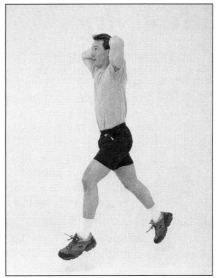

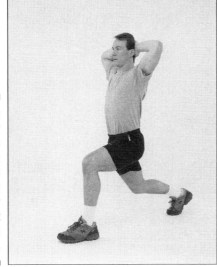

Figure 20-1:
Keep your legs wide apart as you land, and make sure to let your whole foot touch the ground.

Lateral Hop

Although you're not Superman (or -woman), you may feel like it as you hop side to side during this move (see Figure 20-2). For a little adrenalin surge, pretend you're dodging bullets! Make sure to keep controlled and pay attention to your knees. If they feel stressed, stop the move.

Muscles worked: Gluteals, hamstrings, adductors, quadriceps, and calves.

1. **Stand with your feet hip-width apart, and face your toes forward. Place your hands behind your head. Bend your left knee slightly so that you're in a semi-squat position. Push your pelvis out behind you to avoid putting too much forward stress in your bent knee. Extend your right leg.**

2. **Lower your hips slightly and jump up slightly. Shift your body weight to the right foot, keeping the right knee slightly bent as you land. Land softly and with as little jarring to the knee as possible.**

3. **Hold, and then leap to the other side. Repeat.**

Focus & Connect: Think of making a quick weight shift from side to side.

Safety Tip: Keep your jump low and land like a feather.

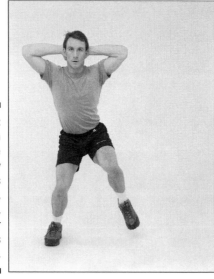

Figure 20-2:
You can improve your agility for sports like tennis, basketball, and soccer with this move.

Slalom Jump Twist

You'll be able to twist the day away on the ski slopes, or during sports that require quick direction changes, if you practice this move (see Figure 20-3).

Muscles worked: Quadriceps, hamstrings, gluteals, abdominals, inner thighs, and erector spinae.

1. **Start with your feet parallel and hip-width apart. First, face your body directly forward. If you're in a room, face one wall. Then shift toward the left corner by twisting yourself to the left a few inches. Your toes, knees, and hips should face the left corner. Hold your arms in front with hands lightly clenched. Lift your ribs, and keep your chest facing forward throughout.**

2. **Jump up and twist your lower body to the right corner. When you land, try not to bend the knees too deeply. Make sure your heels absorb most of your body weight. Repeat.**

Focus & Connect: Simulate a skiing motion and move your lower body as a unit.

Safety Tip: Start with just a slight twist, and then work your way up to a more extreme angle as you get stronger.

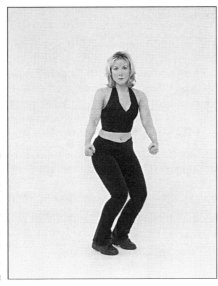 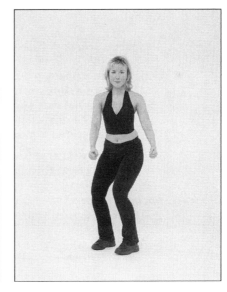

Figure 20-3: Contract your abs to keep your torso stable as you jump and turn.

Calf Toe Run

You may never need to tiptoe through the tulips, but you might be thrown off balance while trying to spike a volleyball or stretching to make a backhand tennis shot and need to get right back on your feet again for the next play. This move helps you develop a little balance and foot control.

Muscles worked: Gastrocnemius, hamstrings, soleus, and quadriceps.

1. **Rise up on your tiptoes and run across 15 feet, or 5 yards.**

2. **Walk back on your heels with your toes up.**

3. **Repeat.**

Focus & Connect: Keep your feet hip-width apart, and think of making yourself as stable as you can.

Safety Tip: Avoid slouching. Keep your upper body tall throughout.

Mountain Climber

Okay, so you may not really want to scale the peaks, but this move lets you pretend. You'll get a little calorie-burning leg action in while developing strength in your core torso muscles.

Muscles worked: Pectorals, triceps, abdominals, and thighs.

1. **Start in a push-up position on your hands with fingers forward and your arms shoulder-width apart. Extend your legs straight behind you, and balance your body weight on your toes. Walk your hands toward the direction of your feet a few inches so your body is in a slight inverted V position, with your hips above the thighs.**

2. **Scissors your feet back and forth quickly as if you were running. Hold your abs tight throughout and drop your head to relax your neck.**

Focus & Connect: Avoid bearing all the weight in your hands. Shift your body weight toward your torso so that you stay evenly balanced.

Safety Tip: If your wrists or back hurt, raise your upper body by leaning against a chair seat or table.

Burst Jump

You can test agility, power, and coordination in this move (see Figure 20-4). However, this is another plyometric jump, so unless you're fit enough to do it and need to improve your explosive ability for a specific sport, you should not do this.

Muscles worked: Quadriceps, calves, hamstrings, gluteals, inner thighs, and abdominals.

1. **Start from the ground. Make sure you're on a soft surface: gym mat, sprung wood floor, or soft ground. Place your feet hip-width apart with toes facing forward, pointing to a low bench. Keep your hands by your sides, knees soft, and back straight. Lean slightly forward.**

2. **Swing your arms back and lower your hips slightly.**

3. **As your arms swing forward, squeeze your glutes and push up off your thighs to jump onto the bench.**

4. **Rather than landing completely, touch down, and then jump straight back onto the ground. Land like a feather. Try not to move faster than you're ready to during this move, because one slipped step and you'll fall. Position most of your foot on the bench each time and pause slightly between up and down phases of the jump if you feel uncontrolled.**

Focus & Connect: Think of your body as a compact, shock-absorbing unit. Touch gently at all points of contact.

Safety Tip: Lift your body upon landing to minimize pounding stress on knees, back, and feet.

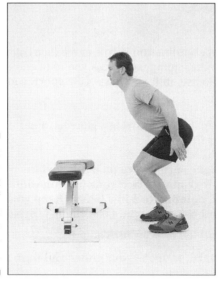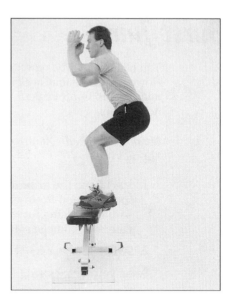

Figure 20-4: Keep the movement controlled if you perform this high-risk plyometric jump.

Depth Jump

You may not have jumped off anything since you were a kid, and if so, you probably shouldn't do this move (see Figure 20-5). It's a tough plyometric exercise where you jump, land, and explode into another jump — not easy for the weary or weak. But if you participate in a sport that requires you to jump and bound and you've already reached a good level of strength, power, and endurance, you may find this move helpful.

Muscles worked: Quadriceps, calves, hamstrings, gluteals, inner thighs, abdominals, and so on.

Before attempting to jump off a platform, start by practicing this move by jumping on soft ground, a gym mat, or a sprung wood floor. Do this for 4-6 weeks before increasing the jump height. Then move up in increments of 2-4 inches. When you've reached the point where you can jump off a high base, don't go any higher than two feet.

1. **In this move, stand on a soft gym mat surface, on soft ground, or on top of a low bench.**

2. **Jump up in the air and back onto the ground.**

3. **Land on both feet in a slight squat and without hesitation explode up in a vertical jump immediately upon landing. Swing your arms upward for added momentum.**

Focus & Connect: To decrease the magnitude of your landing forces, visualize yourself performing a feather light landing. Try not to pound.

Safety Tip: If you feel any discomfort upon landing in your feet, ankles, knees, hips, or back, discontinue this move.

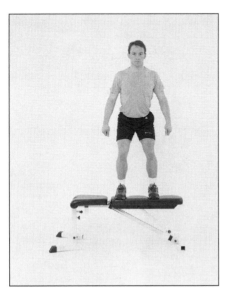
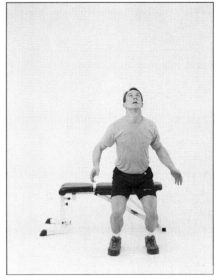
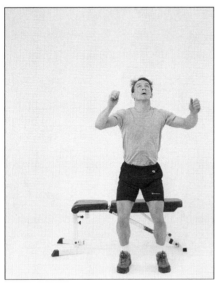

Figure 20-5:
A plyometric jump can improve performance in some sports, but it should not be done unless you are in excellent shape and have no joint injuries.

Chapter 21

Fast, Tricky Moves

• •

In This Chapter

▶ Following agility drills

▶ Getting up to speed

▶ Feeling coordinated

▶ Building strength

• •

*A*ll the strength in the world can't help you if you're not able to carry your own weight around swiftly and nimbly. And, as you'll discover as you plod around the first few times you do these drills, the graceful motions of a champion athlete running for a touchdown, or a dancer performing a series of quick leaps and turns, are a learned skill: what looks easy usually isn't. The good news is that you only have to feel like a klutz at first. With practice you'll be running, leaping, twisting, and turning with the best of them!

To eliminate any potential obstacles during these moves, always check the field or surface you will run or jump on for potholes, uneven spots, and the like. Wear running shoes and make sure that they are in good shock-absorbing condition (they shouldn't be over six months old) and double-tie your shoelaces. In some drills you'll need to mark predetermined spots on the ground. You can use cones, or any other sort of identifier to designate your chosen spots.

Avoid starting at full speed. As you should before beginning any exercise session, warm up first. You can walk through the drills, then gradually jog through them slowly for at least 5-10 minutes. Err on the longer side for your warm up since the exercises will be extremely vigorous. Stretch all your major muscles after warming up and at the end of your workout. When you get down to doing the drills, follow your feelings — if you find the pace to be extremely difficult, slow down. These drills are meant to stimulate, not annihilate, your nervous system. If you feel uncomfortable in any part of your body, slow down or modify the drill. Try not to push yourself to exhaustion, which is easy to do because you'll try to run all-out when aiming for speed. You don't have to sprint if you feel challenged by doing a faster-than-normal jog. Work up to higher intensity workouts gradually.

These drills are hard and fast. For that reason, you won't be spending hours doing them. Start by spending 2-5 minutes on each drill, and work up to 15-20 minutes max, always resting in between repetitions. These are all sports-specific exercises meant to mimic the movements you do in different sports. In most sports, however, you would perform these types of quick bursts of speed, sudden turns, or quick jumps in split-seconds or minute-long intervals. So you shouldn't approach these like you would the typical cardio workout where you might plod along for 45 minutes.

Perform these drills using the *interval* method. After warming up, do a *work interval* of one repetition of your chosen drill for 15-90 seconds. You'll be out of breath and wanting a rest afterwards, so slow down with a *recovery interval* where you walk for 2-5 minutes before repeating another work interval. The less fit you are, the more important it is for you to spend more time on recovery intervals and less time on the work intervals. Avoid stopping still completely during a recovery interval because your body will be in high-intensity work mode. A sudden stop could make you feel more uncomfortable and tired than if you simply slowed down. On your mark, get set, GO!

Straight-Line Cone Drills

Imagine yourself running faster than the speed of light and quicker than the speed of sound! You can do precisely that in this speed drill (or at least try!). You won't turn into Superman (or -woman) the first time out, but after 6-10 weeks of practicing this drill, where you run as fast as you can from one cone marker to the next, you'll definitely increase your race pace.

1. **Place two cones or other visible land markers in a straight line 15 yards apart, as shown in Figure 21-1.**

2. **Stand slightly behind the first cone. Start in either a standing position or a traditional sprinting position.**

   If you decide to go with the standing position, place your feet hip-width apart with your knees slightly bent. Shift your body weight slightly forward. For a traditional sprinting position, crouch in a semi-squat position with your feet hip-width apart. Place your stronger leg slightly in front of the other, and place one or both hands — fingers down — on the ground in front of you.

3. **Explode forward into a sprint by pushing off the ground with your front, or stronger leg.**

4. **Sprint to the second cone at full speed and run past it, stopping afterwards, rather than slowing your pace in order to stop right at the cone.**

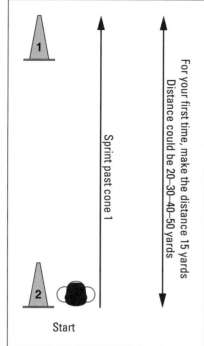

Figure 21-1:
Place the cones 15 yards apart for your first time. Once you're familiar with the drill and feel comfortable sprinting, you can add more distance and eventually add more cones (see the Advanced option).

For your first time, make the distance 15 yards
Distance could be 20–30–40–50 yards

Sprint past cone 1

1

2

Start

Advanced option: Once you feel comfortable with this drill, increase the space between the cones to 20, 30, 40, and 50 yards. Then, when you reach 50 yards, place two more cones in the middle of the original two and sprint from cone 1 to 2, then lightly jog from cone 2 to 3, then sprint from cone 3 to 4, and then lightly jog back to the beginning cone.

Focus & Connect: Feel the power in your thighs as you run.

Safety Tip: Avoid stopping too suddenly; slow down gradually.

Square Cone Drill

If you're an ex–high school or –grade school athlete and miss the rigours of sports practice, you can take a jog down memory lane with this cone drill that has you shuffling forward and from side to side as quickly as you can. This tests your ability to make quick stops, turns, and sprints — skills you'll need during a high-charged football, soccer, basketball, or even tennis game. You'll improve your speed and balance by doing this exercise regularly.

1. **Place four cones in a square, five yards apart from each other (see Figure 21-2).**

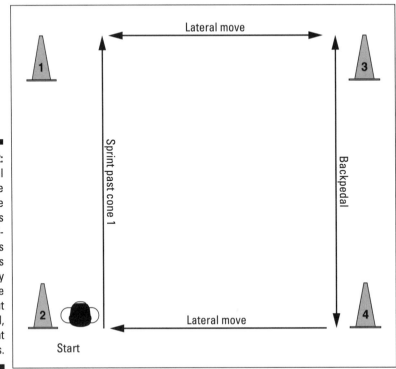

Figure 21-2:
The lateral move in the square cone drill tests your balance skills as well as your ability to move quickly, but with control, in different directions.

2. **Staying on the inside of the cones, run from cone 1 to cone 2 — touch each cone you reach. Then shuffle fast laterally from cone 2 to cone 3 and use your peripheral vision to determine your stopping point. Backpedal from cone 3 to cone 4, and then shuffle to cone 1 again. Repeat.**

Focus & Connect: Think of your body as a compact unit throughout the pattern.

Safety Tip: Avoid coming to a jarring stop when you reach a cone: Run past it or stop gradually before.

In-and-Out Cone Drill

Grab your running shoes (or even your inline skates if you do the drill on pavement instead of grass), and weave in and out of a set of cones. During a competitive activity or sport you may have to be able to roll with the punches, or rather, deal with the continually changing circumstances of the game. If someone is coming at you, you need to dodge out of the way. If you're chasing after something (a ball) or someone (a big, fast guy) that's moving erratically, you need to be able to shift your weight, speed up and slow down, and duck and dodge. This move has you mimic these movement patterns to develop agility and speed.

1. **Place nine cones in a zigzag line, staggered three to four yards apart from each other (see Figure 21-3).**

   If you don't have the resources, you can substitute the nine cones for just four. Follow the same directions.

2. **Weave in and out around the top and bottom of the cones. Jog backward (backpedal) from cone 1 to cone 2; from cone 2 to cone 3, sprint forward. Follow this backpedal and sprint pattern until you pass all the cones. When nearing the last cone, sprint past it.**

Focus & Connect: Take shorter, rather than longer, steps.

Safety Tip: When you change directions, switch your starting foot. So to move right, lead with the right foot. To move left, lead with the left foot.

Lateral Cone Drill

Do the shuffle. You won't have music, but you can shake your booty down to the ground and block anything or anyone that dares try to get past you if you do this drill often enough! Whether you're a soccer goalie, a tennis or softball player trying to stop a ball from going past you, or a football or basketball player trying to make sure no one else advances, you'll need to be able to move sideways *fast*. This move will help you develop balance to accommodate quick shifts in direction. You'll also improve your overall speed and coordination.

1. **Place two cones 10 yards apart in a horizontal line, as shown in Figure 21-4.**

2. **Start in a semi-squat position behind and slightly inside cone 1. Touch the cone with your outside hand.**

3. **Shuffle laterally as fast as you can, moving toward cone 2 while crossing your feet back and forth. To move toward the right, step with the outside right foot and alternate crossing your left foot in front of the right; step right again and cross your left foot behind the right. Step out again. Continue and pick up the pace once you have the foot pattern down.**

4. **Touch the cone with your outside hand and reverse the movement.**

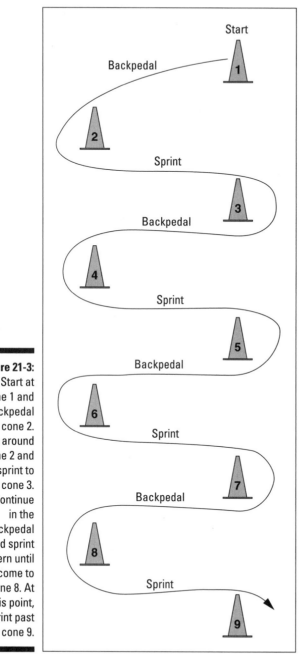

Figure 21-3:
Start at
cone 1 and
backpedal
to cone 2.
Go around
cone 2 and
sprint to
cone 3.
Continue
in the
backpedal
and sprint
pattern until
you come to
cone 8. At
this point,
sprint past
cone 9.

Focus & Connect: Pick up your feet and think of making a choppy but fluid sideways motion as you travel.

Safety Tip: If you have unstable ankles, work on improving your balance by doing such moves as the single leg extension or standing side leg lift in Chapter 17 before adding speed to your foot patterns.

Figure 21-4:
First concentrate on executing the crossover foot pattern with control. Then concentrate on speed.

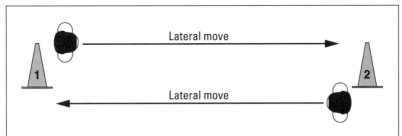

Zigzag Drill

"Keep your eye on the ball" is one of the golden rules of sport that you no doubt have heard whether you've played golf, tennis, basketball, or baseball. Whether you're catching, hitting, throwing, or kicking, your ability to stay focused on your target is the key to success. The tricky part is that the ball doesn't usually come to you; you usually have to go to it. This means that you often have to look in a completely different direction than you're moving. If you're a receiver in football, you have to run in a designated pattern with your eye focused on the quarterback. This skill requires you to be able to have enough body awareness to move quickly in ever-changing directions, without being able to fully focus on looking where you're going. This drill has you twisting and turning while looking the other way. You'll improve your balance, agility, and body awareness by practicing it.

1. **Place six cones in a zigzag line with each cone 5-10 yards apart, as shown in Figure 21-5.**

   Three cones should form a line on the right, and three cones should form a parallel line on the left, with the left cones placed at the midpoint between the cones on the right.

2. **Sprint from the starting cone 1 to cone 2 while keeping your eye on cone 1 (your head should be turned back toward your right). Sprint from cone 2 toward cone 3 (which is on the left), keeping your eyes on cone 1. Sprint toward cone 4 with head turned right and eye on cone 1. Then sprint toward cone 5 with your head turned left and eye on cone 1. Finally, sprint toward cone 6 with your head turned right and eye on cone 1.**

3. **From cone 6, follow the same drill to return to cone 1.**

Focus & Connect: Stay in a low athletic position during sprints to allow you to stop, start, and shift body weight quickly and with ease.

Safety Tip: If you feel unstable — rather than risk twisting an ankle, knee, or your lower back during the quick changes — slow your traveling steps and focus on your form and balance with your head turned.

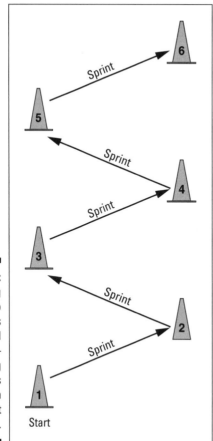

Figure 21-5:
In the zigzag drill, keep your eyes on a fixed point — your starting cone — as you run in different directions.

Horseshoe Drill

Advance-and-retreat is the underlying pattern found in most competitive sports. You need to be able to perform all out bursts forward (to chase someone or something), but then be able to stop quickly and move backward with control (to get away from a charging opponent, or reposition yourself to catch a throw). This drill helps develop your forward/back movement responses. You'll develop speed, agility, and control over your footsteps.

1. **Arrange six cones in a diamond shape, as shown in Figure 21-6.**

   The four points on the diamond are five yards apart. Place a starting cone at the lowest point. Cone 1 is at the left point, cone 3 is at the top point, and cone 5 is at the right point. Cone 2 is midway between cone 1 and 3. Cone 4 is midway between cone 3 and 5.

2. **Begin at the starting cone, and burst forward and run to cone 1.**

3. **Jog backward to cone 1 again.**

4. **Burst forward to cone 2, and backpedal to the starting cone again.**

5. **Run from the starting cone to cone 3 and back, from the starting cone to cone 4 and back, and from the starting cone to cone 5 and back.**

Focus & Connect: Try to establish a rhythm to your bursts of speed.

Safety Tip: If your knees hurt from the forward sprints, slow down your pace.

Grass-Drop Drill

It's not just your legs that need to be able to perform explosive action during sports, but your upper body as well. Since many sports have lots of spills and tumbles, when you're under the gun and the clock is ticking, you need to be able to pop back up to score that winning goal or throw the ball to home plate. This move uses your body weight as your main method of resistance. You'll pretend you're in the heat of the moment by running in place, then you'll drop to the ground and raise yourself back up again. You'll develop agility, power, and strength from practicing this move.

1. **Start in a ready stance: a semi-squat position, body weight shifted slightly forward, and hands in front of your thighs.**

2. **Run in place as quickly as you can for three seconds (count *one thousand one, one thousand two, one thousand three*).**

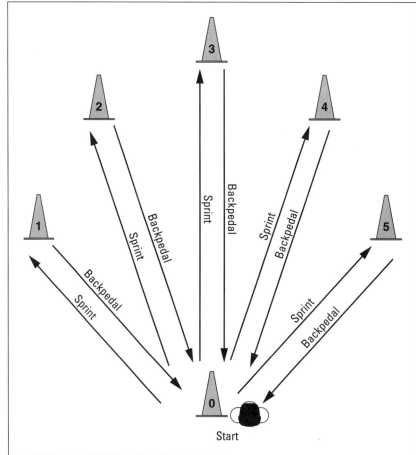

Figure 21-6:
Just think "Charge!" as you burst toward each cone. Then think "Whoa" and backtrack to your starting position.

3. **Drop to the ground on your forearm, abs, and front thighs (legs outstretched behind you). Hold your chest high and look forward.**

4. **Explode up to a standing position quickly.**

5. **Jog again, drop, and jump up. Repeat.**

Focus & Connect: Feel buoyant as you use your thighs and glutes to spring up and down.

Safety Tip: Give your bony parts a little tender-loving care and practice this drill on a soft surface like grass or a gym mat — remember it's not called the concrete-drop drill!

Dancer's Leap

Sports aren't the only activities that require Herculean efforts. In daily life, you might find it necessary to make an Olympic leap over a mud puddle or a quick jump to dodge an oncoming bike, skater, or car. This move simulates a skip, hop, and a jump with the grace of a dancer's approach. It's almost an elongated run; you move forward with your legs reaching farther and your body lifting higher with each step. Because a leg stretch is part of the split-leg action, you'll be developing some dynamic flexibility or stretching while moving. You need to be warm and supple enough to do this maneuver, so spend a little more time on your warm up and preworkout stretch before doing it. You might also find that the lunge scissor kick in Chapter 18 is a helpful exercise to complement your performance of this move.

1. **Find a field or room where you can travel at least 15 yards. Start with your feet shoulder-width apart, hands by your sides.**

2. **Leap and travel forward while swinging your arms in opposition to your legs. Jump and simultaneously extend your right leg forward in the air in a split position and extend and raise the left leg in back. Let your left arm swing forward with the right foot to help you glide through the air.**

3. **Land gently, and then switch: Right arm swings forward as your left leg kicks forward. Repeat and make the traveling motion as fluid as possible.**

Focus & Connect: Stay low as you travel, but aim to cover as much space as possible per leap.

Safety Tip: Keep your legs close together if your hamstrings are tight, or if you're especially inflexible. Always warm up and stretch before this drill.

Bunny Hops

Nothing beats a good jump, which must explain why people winning the lottery feel the urge to burst up in a big emotional moment, or why groups of drunken people at weddings spontaneously group into a line of wobbly hoppers when the right song comes along. Jumping is a powerful, high-impact movement — but one that you'll use in almost every sport from hopscotch to basketball. Technically, there are jumps, hops, and leaps, where you transfer your body weight in an explosive moment from point A to point B while on both feet, one foot, or from foot-to-opposite foot. This drill incorporates all three variations and will help improve your reflexes and will help you develop quick, explosive leg power.

1. Create a 10-yard line by spreading out a jump rope on the grass, or find a line on a track or field you can use.

2. Stand on the left side of the line with your feet parallel and knees slightly bent.

3. Jump forward on and off both feet at once in a zigzag pattern over the line — alternate your touchdown points on either side of the line. Jump quickly and touch down toes-only as briefly as possible at the midpoints.

4. When you get to the end of the line, land completely on your heels.

5. Repeat the pattern hopping on one foot, and then switching to the other foot. Repeat leaping from one foot to another.

Focus & Connect: Aim to stay off the ground throughout most of the journey from the beginning to endpoint.

Safety Tip: If the impact of the jumps feels too stressful on your feet or legs when you land, jump more slowly and slightly lower, allowing your heels to touch down each time. Always find a soft surface — dirt, grass, sprung-wood floor, or soft track — on which to jump.

Part V
Move That Body!

The 5th Wave   By Rich Tennant

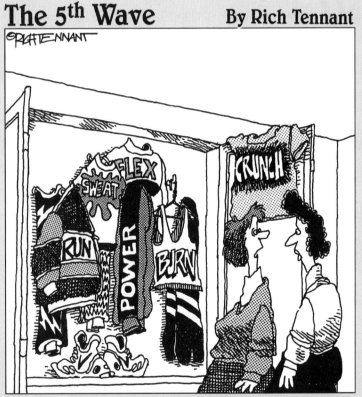

"I'm not sure I can live up to my workout clothes."

In this part . . .

You get to consider all the possibilities, all the paths you can take in your cross-training life. We run down the most common solo sports like running and inline skating, highlight the key things you should know about the activity, and point out training techniques and exercises that will help improve your performance. In the middle chapter, we outline the different types of fitness classes available and what to expect if you take them. The final chapter discusses team sports — different ways to train to improve your fitness and skill levels, as well as key things to do to maintain overall balance in your body. Look up the activities you already participate in, and check to see if you're training in the right way.

When trying any new activity, remember to take it slow. Don't assume that just because you're fit at another activity, your body is ready to plunge full-force into an intense session of something new — it's not.

Chapter 22

The Solo Sporting Life

In This Chapter

▶ Different activities you can do by yourself

▶ Key training tips for walking, running, skating, hiking, and swimming

▶ The mothersport of all cross-training: triathlons

Some of the most effective activities are also the most accessible. We highlight the top seven types of cardio workouts that you can do on your own, almost anywhere that you may live. You can do these without a teammate and with a minimal amount of equipment. They can be a source of solitary pleasure, or you can get competitive and enter race events. We also tell you more about triathlons, one of the true cross-training sports since they incorporate running, cycling, and swimming.

Walking

Walking is not only one of the most economical and hassle-free activities you can do, it's a great way to sneak exercise in to your daily life. It is generally low to moderate intensity and emphasizes cardio stamina. If you do it fast enough and long enough, it can also be a good way to blast calories.

Because your body is pretty used to it, you'll have to walk briskly for an extended period of time to feel the effects. To up the ante, alternate short and long strides to pick up the pace. Avoid using light hand weights. Hand weights seem like a good idea, but in fact, they won't help you burn many more calories or improve your arm and shoulder strength. Studies have shown that they don't increase intensity much and could lead to injuries in your shoulders.

To mix things up, try walking in sand, in water, on trails, on the treadmill, with your dog, or in the shopping mall. Hiking is another variation you may want to try.

Pros and cons

Walking is a good place to start when you're new to exercise. You can do it inside on a treadmill or outside, no matter where you are. Although you can improve your cardio stamina, since it's easier to stroll rather than to power-walk, you have to make sure to push yourself to jack up the intensity of a walking workout.

What you need to know

Walking shoes will make a tremendous difference if you're going to walk for long periods. Perfect your walking technique; step and land with your heel, ball, and then toe. Pump your arms in opposition to your legs, but try not to clench your fists. As you walk along, keep your chin up — instead of looking down at your feet — and pay attention to the path a few yards ahead.

If you walk a lot, you may feel soreness in the front of your shin. This is from the foot lifting up repetitively with each step. As your muscles get used to the exertion, the pain will subside. You can help strengthen the anterior tibialis and other lower leg muscles with the toe tap exercise — while standing, simply lift one toe up and down, keeping your heel on the ground. Repeat 30 times on each foot. Try our foot and ankle stretch in Chapter 15 to stretch out this area when it gets tight.

Recommended training, cross-training, and stretches

Increase your speed by taking shorter, faster strides. When going uphill, take longer strides. Move your arms in sync with your steps, and keep your elbows at approximately 90 degrees and close to your body.

You can add weight training, rowing, dancing, and skills drills (see Chapter 21) to your program as cross-training activities.

You should always warm up and stretch all major muscles, but be sure to spend a little extra time on the following muscle groups that can get over-worked in this activity. Check out Chapters 15 and 28 for exercises to loosen up your hamstrings, hip, torso, and calves (the calves are part of the muscle group that includes the soleus).

To improve your posture and walking technique, include these exercises as part of your regular training program:

✔ Squats (see Chapter 16)

✔ Back lunges (see Chapter 16)

✔ Back extensions (see Chapter 17)

✔ Standing side leg lifts (see Chapter 17)

Running

Forrest Gump never stopped, and neither should you. Even though running is a regular part of childhood, for some reason, once we grow up we get lazy and then find it too difficult to do something as natural as run. Running is great for building cardio stamina and muscular endurance, especially in the legs, and plays a part in almost every sport except for golf, snow and water sports, and surfing the Web. But it's also a high-intensity activity that can be unnecessarily stressful if you push too hard too soon or try to do it too often. You can also do damage if you run despite body weaknesses, such as joint injuries that can be aggravated by the high impact.

The body was born to run and for most running is perfectly safe, provided you wear proper running shoes, stick to mostly soft surfaces (running track or a shock-absorbing treadmill as opposed to concrete), keep each session short, and limit the frequency to no more than three to five runs per week if you're extremely fit and healthy, and less if you're a beginning runner. Long distance training, like marathon training, increases the likelihood of overuse injuries from wear and tear. If you're going to run long distances, do it properly. Approach it like you'd approach any other cross-training plan: Build up a base with shorter distance jogs, or even walks of two to three miles to prepare your body for the extra speed, distances, and sessions.

The belief before the 1960s was that running was dangerous for women because it jostled all their internal bits around. Provided a woman has no joint problems, has strong and healthy pelvic floor muscles, and is fit enough to do it, running is a great form of exercise.

To vary your running routine, try trail running or water running with a flotation device. You can also vary your workout with Fartlek training, where you pick a point in the distance and run as fast as you can, then run slower for a recovery interval, and then continue to alternate the fast and slower pace. If the competitive edge overtakes you, enter some short fun runs or 5/10k races. If you have the time to train for it, try a marathon where you run 26.2 miles.

Pros and cons

Running is one of the most time-efficient ways to exercise. If you're fit enough and have a short amount of time, running can give you the most bang for your buck when it comes to burning calories and increasing cardio stamina. You can do it alone, you can do it with a friend, or you can join thousands of like-minded people in races.

Unfortunately, running is a high-impact activity. If you're stuck doing it on sidewalks and roads, your joints may not enjoy long sessions. If you feel any aches and pains, listen to your body and modify your fitness program accordingly. Runners are notorious for ignoring body signs that point to running too much — until it's too late and they're stuck with chronic injuries.

What you need to know

If you start running, you can get hooked, which is a good thing, unless you do it too hard, too long, or too often. Then you'll start to feel all those aches that are so common in so many runners.

Also, avoid running with a portable stereo blasting in your ears. You can risk eardrum damage and not being able to hear oncoming traffic or suspicious people if you're running alone.

To avoid running injuries, learn to run with perfect form. Analyze the runners in front of you on your daily jog. Notice the different gaits and postures. Notice how some people run in a very compact, controlled fashion; others seem to splay their limbs everywhere. Notice the different stride lengths and spinal alignments: Some people hunch forward, round their shoulders, and look at the ground, while others lean to one side or shift their bodies excessively side to side. Some people shuffle, their feet barely lifting the ground, and others throw their feet up and swing them around, almost out to the side before they land again. Imbalances in the way that people hold their bodies can exacerbate the stress on the back, hips, knees, and feet when they run.

Notice the foot width of different body types during each stride. The ideal runner has small hips and his feet are consistently stacked beneath his hips with each step.

All of the potential body imbalances play a key role in running injuries. Pay special attention to correcting your own running flaws. Here are a few tips:

- ✔ Keep your hips, shoulders, knees, and feet stacked.
- ✔ Avoid twisting your torso with each step.
- ✔ Look forward, not down.
- ✔ Lower your shoulders and lift your rib cage.
- ✔ Land softly with each step.

Recommended training, cross-training, and stretches

For basic training, alternate longer runs and shorter, faster runs to vary the stresses on your body. Stretch regularly. Use cycling and aqua jogging with a flotation belt or vest to improve leg endurance while minimizing the impact. Also incorporate swimming, martial arts, and an active rest activity, such as Ping-Pong, into your cross-training program.

You should always warm up and stretch all major muscles, but be sure to spend a little extra time on the following muscle groups that can get over-worked in this activity. Check out Chapters 15 and 28 for exercises to loosen up your soleus, quadriceps, hamstrings, calves, and buttocks.

To enhance your running performance, include these exercises as part of your regular training program:

- ✔ Weighted walking lunges (see Chapter 18)
- ✔ Jump lunges (see Chapter 20)
- ✔ Back extensions (see Chapter 17)
- ✔ Military presses overhead (see Chapter 17)
- ✔ Lat pulldowns (see Chapter 19)

Hiking

A meander through the forest will lift just about anyone's spirit. Hiking is another term for rugged walking off-road. Since you're bound to run across lots of bumps, holes, stumps, lumps, and logs, you'll need special hiking boots that have better traction than ordinary walking shoes.

Hiking really emphasizes cardio stamina, agility, endurance, lower body strength, balance, and upper body strength (if you carry a backpack).

Pros and cons

A hike is a great butt and leg workout, and it burns more calories than a regular walk, especially if you're on hilly terrain. But you also increase your likelihood of stumbles, trips, and twisted ankles because you have to constantly avoid holes and stumps. Depending upon how far out you go, you need to know how to protect yourself in the wilderness.

What you need to know

Follow the Boy Scouts motto and "Be prepared." It's better to be overprepared when it comes to trampling around in the wilderness. Bring a first-aid kit, bug spray, a blanket, extra water, and food. Wear bright clothes so you can be seen. Stay on marked paths.

Go slow. When you're carrying an extra 30 pounds up steep paths for several hours, you're getting a very intensive workout that you might not be aware of unless you stop suddenly and notice how fast your heart is beating. The environment around you helps distract you from fatigue. You need your strength since you never know what big hill, big hole, or big critter is around the corner.

Also, if you're walking in high altitudes, you might find it more difficult because the change in oxygen levels can leave you short of breath if you're not used to it.

Recommended training, cross-training, and stretches

To prepare for wilderness walks, include upper body weight exercises to help train for spending hours carrying a backpack and also include lower body strength work. You might want to include bowling and other activities that hone your balance.

You should always warm up and stretch all major muscles, but be sure to spend a little extra time on the following muscle groups that can get overworked in this activity. Check out Chapters 15 and 28 for exercises to loosen up your soleus, quadriceps, hamstrings, calves, and buttocks.

Include the following exercises into your preparation sessions to get you strong for the trail:

- ✔ Back lunges (see Chapter 16)
- ✔ Triceps kickbacks (see Chapter 17)
- ✔ Dynamic side lunges (see Chapter 18)
- ✔ Single leg extensions (see Chapter 17)
- ✔ Lunge scissor kicks (see Chapter 18)

Cycling Outside

Riding a bike can be as easy or as hard as you make it. The joy of cycling outside is that it doesn't feel much like exercise, except of course if you're climbing hills or sprinting.

Cycling really tests your cardiovascular and muscular endurance in the lower body. Your lower body will need power to push you through those upcoming hills, and you need to utilize balance and agility to maneuver your bike.

If the weather outside is icky, you can try indoor cycling classes (called *Spinning* classes) and stationary biking. If you're into a challenge, try mountain biking, racing, triathlons, or biathlons.

Pros and cons

Cycling is low impact and easy to do. Unfortunately, cycling can get very expensive if you go for the custom-made bike with a titanium frame and so on. And, it can be high risk if you're on roads with cars.

What you need to know

You must wear a helmet. Sometimes beginners feel a little stupid with them on because they think it makes them look like a beginner. In fact, if you notice all the serious cyclists in packs wearing their colorful gear, they're all wearing helmets because they know they'd be stupid not to. Helmets have protected a lot of lives. Don't look like a beginner and go cycling without one.

It's not just your legs that get a workout. You can get a sore butt and tired feet from long sessions on a bike. Four key tools can help alleviate your discomfort:

 ✔ Get proper cycling shoes instead of wearing your workout shoes. These have a firm sole, which means that your foot muscles don't have to work so hard to push the pedal around.

 ✔ Try toe clips on your pedals. Many beginners are afraid that their feet will get trapped during a fall. You can choose from several types of toe clips, the simplest of which is a curved piece of plastic attached to the top of a pedal that covers only the toe of your shoe. Once you get used to toe clips, you will be able to insert and remove your foot from them with ease. They will make pedaling and taking control of your bike much easier.

✔ Wear padded bike shorts. It's amazing what an extra layer of padding can do for a sore behind. You can choose from different styles of bike shorts and pants that have specially inserted chamois padding from crotch to rear.

✔ Try a wider bicycle seat. Traditionally seats have been thin, hard, and very uncomfortable, especially for women. But now many female-friendly versions of bike seats are available. They redistribute the seat pressure so that it doesn't all concentrate on your private parts. Over a long ride, it will make a difference.

Recommended training, cross-training, and stretches

Include leg strength moves and back extension exercises to counterattack the forward lean of riding a bike. Keep your upper body strong with strength exercises, and train for the upper body with the rowing machine, upper body ergometer, and the Versiclimber.

You can cross-train by playing sports or taking group fitness classes. Agility drills can help develop coordination that you may be missing out from cycling-only workouts.

You should always warm up and stretch all major muscles, but be sure to spend a little extra time on the following muscle groups that can get overworked in this activity. Check out Chapters 15 and 28 for exercises to loosen up your quads, hips, hamstrings, gluteals, and calves before venturing on the open road.

Try these exercises to improve your cycling performance:

✔ Back lunges (see Chapter 16)

✔ Single leg extensions (see Chapter 17)

✔ Back extensions (see Chapter 17)

✔ Rubber band rows (see Chapter 17)

Inline Skating

Not many new sports have taken the population by storm, but inline skating has. This cool activity revived what was once only a childhood pastime. Inline skates are so-called because the wheels run in a single line, much like an ice skate, as opposed to the square formation of four-wheeled roller skates. Skating gives a great total body workout and, best of all, the time just whizzes by.

Inline skating focuses on lower body muscular endurance and power, cardio stamina, balance, and agility.

A few variations of this popular sport are skating outside on roads or park paths, skating in roller rinks, skating on ice rinks, playing roller hockey, skating distance events, and performing skating tricks.

Pros and cons

Even though it's a very intense exercise, it feels easy because it's so much fun. Unfortunately, skating can be high risk if you don't take precautions. Make sure you can go down a steep hill with your breaks on before attempting to skate on hilly paths. You can take an inline skating class, or even have a session with an inline skating personal trainer for basic technique when you first start out.

What you need to know

Stick to smooth surfaces; avoid gravel, sticks, and slick spots. Always wear pads and a helmet: Pads should cover your wrists, elbows, and knees. To date a butt pad hasn't been invented, but that's okay because most of the time you fall forward!

Your key to success is learning how to stop before you learn how to do anything else. Different skates have different brake systems, but generally you stop by sliding your brake foot forward and lowering your body weight on the heel to lift the toe slightly (and drag the brake on the ground). Remember that you will never stop abruptly on skates (unless you intend to follow the stop with a somersault). You will gradually come to a stop by slowing your speed down. So plan your stops in advance and gauge your speed by how much stopping distance you may need.

Recommended training, cross-training, and stretches

To get in good skating shape, include lower body strength and power exercises as well as agility drills into your training plan. To cross-train, add upper body strength moves and activities that require more coordination such as basketball and tennis.

You should always warm up and stretch all major muscles, but be sure to spend a little extra time on the following muscle groups that can get over-worked in this activity. Check out Chapters 15 and 28 for exercises to loosen up your hamstrings, gluteals, quads, and inner thighs before hitting the pavement.

Include the following exercises into your training sessions to improve your performance:

✔ Back extensions (see Chapter 17)

✔ Standing side leg lifts (see Chapter 17)

✔ Military presses overhead (see Chapter 17)

✔ Lateral raises (see Chapter 17)

Rowing

Rowing has a cult-like following, as you can tell from the plethora of films that feature this popular sport. Generally, people new to the sport tend to lump two- and three-man skulling, canoeing, and kayaking under the term rowing. Technically, however, *rowing* refers to the motion you use on an indoor rowing machine or in a canoe when you row with one oar. If you row with two oars, you're sculling. Sculling also uses a sliding seat so that you employ leg power along with each arm stroke. Kayaking involves paddles and a smaller, lighter boat.

Depending on the type of rowing you do (and we're using the term inter-changeably here), it involves more than just arm movement but also the power of your torso and legs to push the oars. You'll notice increased cardio stamina, upper body endurance, core strength, and flexibility.

Pros and cons

Rowing is a great calorie burner, but the sport comes with a lot of negative aspects. The sculling technique is complicated, and it involves a lot of prac-tice on your part to get really good at it. You also need to know how to swim, and you need water and a boat! You can also row indoors on a *rowing ergome-ter,* a nonelectric piece of equipment that most closely simulates the feel of rowing on water, or a rowing machine. The constant torso twist and leaning back and forth can be tough on your back.

What you need to know

You might tip over and lose everything in the boat, especially if you're a beginner, so make sure your watch and glasses are strapped on and leave your valuables at the boathouse. Wear warm clothing.

Before you can get a good workout rowing, you have to learn how to do it properly. Otherwise, you're so busy trying to balance and keep hold of your oars that you're not going to move very fast. To keep your boat from tipping, never let go of the oars/paddles and never bring your hands behind your body as you row. If you're with others, avoid locking oars with other crew members, relax, and mimic the speed of the person in front of you.

Recommended training, cross-training, and stretches

Row on the stationary boat first, a kind of boatlike treadmill that's anchored in the water. Also, run to help improve leg power and swim to build your swimming skills in case of emergency.

To cross-train, do activities that improve your coordination such as basketball and tennis.

You should always warm up and stretch all major muscles, but be sure to spend a little extra time on the following muscle groups that can get overworked in this activity. Check out Chapters 15 and 28 for exercises to loosen up your hamstrings, torso, back, and gluteals.

These exercises are extra effective for helping you get a strong rowing body:

- ✔ Rubber band rows (see Chapter 17)
- ✔ Back extensions (see Chapter 17)
- ✔ Ab crunches on ball (see Chapter 17)

Swimming

Some people are naturals in the water and feel a special sense of calm from the meditative, in-your-own-world effect of swimming. The world of swimming has many opportunities besides your local swimming hole. You can choose to swim in pools, lakes, or the ocean. Snorkeling and scuba diving appeal to nature lovers, while triathlons, water aerobics, aqua jogging, and aqua step appeal to more disciplined exercisers.

Swimming emphasizes cardio stamina, muscular endurance, and core strength (to keep the body positioned).

Pros and cons

Swimming is very low-impact exercise for most people. However, some swimming strokes can exacerbate knee and back problems, so tread carefully. Overall, swimming is a great total body workout and helps strengthen back and postural muscles as well as the butt and thighs.

However, you need a pool and you need to know how to swim before you can feel the calming and energizing effects of swimming.

What you need to know

Speedos are not required for men. If you're in a competition where every second counts, they'll shave time off your speed. If you don't want to be mistaken for a European or poser bodybuilder by available women, leave your Lycra at home. Triathlon suits and cycling shorts, on the other hand, are almost as revealing, but they have that touch of mystery that women love while still showing off all the right curves.

Take lessons to review your swimming strokes. Long sessions using poor technique can cause overuse injuries in the shoulders, neck, and back.

Recommended training, cross-training, and stretches

To get in shape for swimming, do both upper and lower body strength moves plus exercises that strengthen your core back and ab muscles. Practice kicking drills with kickboards, also called paddleboards, and use resistance cords to train for strength in the water. Aqua resistance tools, such as hand paddles and pull buoys, work your upper body.

You may want to include running and other sports into your cross-training plan.

You should always warm up and stretch all major muscles, but be sure to spend a little extra time on the following muscle groups that can get overworked in this activity. Check out Chapters 15 and 28 for exercises to loosen up your deltoids, back, chest, and gluteals.

Exercises you can do to help strengthen and improve your swimming performance include:

✔ Push-ups (see Chapter 16)

✔ Rotator cuff (see the "Racquet Sports" section in Chapter 24)

✔ Single leg extensions (see Chapter 17)

✔ Back extensions (see Chapter 17)

Triathlons

Triathlons (events where you run, bike, and swim) are cross-training events in action. *Duathlons,* also known as biathlons, are events where you bike and run. The best-known triathlon, the Ironman, requires competitors to swim 2.4 miles, cycle 112 miles, and run a full marathon (26.2 miles) — no mean feat.

Because of the intensity of this sport, be ready to build your cardio stamina, muscular endurance for upper and lower body, power, flexibility, and strength.

Pros and cons

The triathlon is a competitive sport that provides a lot of variety and challenge. You can do them on your own, or train and compete with friends.

The cons of triathlons are training for these events takes time (a lot of it) and access to swimming facilities. Plus, the bike can be expensive.

What you need to know

Since each sport you train for has its own unique requirements, you should read up on how to train for a triathlon and join a local triathlon training group to help you go through the paces. It's a tough endurance activity, and you need to prepare, prepare, prepare.

Recommended training, cross-training, and stretches

Divide your time wisely and work on your weakest link, rather than spending most of your training doing that which comes easiest. When it comes to the race, what will slow you down is your weakness — for most people that's swimming.

Your training must include cycling, running, swimming, upper and lower body strength work, and stretching.

Agility drills, aerobics, yoga, and other sports are great activities for your cross-training plan. These activities will boost your flexibility, power, and agility, making you stronger and more prepared for the big race.

You should always warm up and stretch all major muscles, but be sure to spend a little extra time on the following muscle groups that can get over-worked with these three base sports. Check out Chapters 15 and 28 for exercises to loosen up your quadriceps, hamstrings, back, calves, soleus, adductors, chest, shoulders, and triceps.

Improve your performance by including lunges and upper and lower body strength work. See the "Running," "Cycling Outside," and "Swimming" sections for more detailed suggestions.

Chapter 23

Movin' to the Groove

· ·

In This Chapter

▶ Trying a new fitness class

▶ Introducing the many types of group fitness classes

· ·

*A*erobics classes used to consist of a series of choreographed dance moves done to a groovy disco beat. The participants were mostly women with big hair in thong leotards and matching flop socks. If men dared to enter a class at all, they were Richard Simmons look-alikes. This had a certain appeal for some. Martica was one of them. She has fond memories of taking her first aerobics class in 1982 and seeing a glamorous ensemble of bright pink legwarmers and a pink-and-black striped leotard. Right then she knew that she had to become an aerobics instructor, so she could wear these fabulous outfits full time.

Now, things have changed. Although some fitness fashion victims are still around, you'll also find women in baggy T-shirts, no makeup, and no interest in the dance type of aerobics. These women love the sweat and challenge of boxing-style classes or athletic circuit-training sessions. And guys aren't such a rare commodity anymore, either. You'll find lots of men of all ages, shapes, and sizes, punching, kicking, twisting, and stepping to the beat with the best of them.

Aerobics By Any Other Name

Aerobics has a new name to match its new identity: *group fitness*. Group fitness encompasses the concept that made the original aerobics classes so popular: a group of people exercising to music (usually), led by a motivating instructor. Part of the reason for the name change is that the aerobics phenomenon was misnamed in the first place. The word *aerobic* actually signifies what aerobic dance exercise improves — the aerobic, or cardiovascular, system. And aerobic exercise is more than just dance. Running, cycling, walking, and soccer are also aerobic activities. Group fitness is a more apt description because it doesn't limit what the classes can be.

Aerobics was always stereotyped as a bunch of women, dancing around and doing high kicks and grapevines. In fact, group fitness classes are not all the same, nor do they all incorporate dance moves, nor are they all aerobic.

The beauty of the fitness industry is that all the regulars — from the instructors and personal trainers, down to the fitness disciples who never miss a class — get bored easily, so they're constantly looking for new ways to spice up group fitness classes. What has happened as a result is that there are so many different styles and formats of fitness classes being taught in most health clubs that you could probably try a new type of class every day for a month. If you're someone that's always stuck to the gym and cardio machines, or have never even gotten as far as joining a health club, you'd be surprised at the range of classes that you can try and may even find that you love!

Group fitness classes might contain yoga moves, use dumbbells and barbells, or be taught on a stationary bike. Even the bonafide dance-exercise classes vary immensely — they range from consisting of very funky and highly choreographed MTV-style routines to including simple, athletic, or calisthenic moves that anyone can follow.

So what does this mean to you? It means that no matter how klutzy or unfit you think you might be, you can find a group fitness class you'll feel comfortable doing — and you need never strap on a lycra bodysuit to take one.

We've compiled a list of the most popular classes out there. As part of your cross-training prescription, we recommend that you try at least one, if not several.

Our advice is to try not to pigeonhole yourself as the type who doesn't like — or can't do — fitness classes. Not all classes require coordination. Sculpting, stretching, circuit, and martial arts–based classes usually contain simple moves like you used to do in P.E. (think of jumping jacks and jogging in place). Plus a good instructor makes everyone in the class feel comfortable, by breaking down exercises and routines so that everyone can follow, by giving good technique tips so that you feel confident about the way you're doing a move, and by modifying moves that might not be right for everyone in the class. If you try a class and don't have a comfortable experience, chances are the instructor is not very good. Don't give up; try a few more classes with different teachers.

What You Should Know When Trying a Group Fitness Class

If the fear-of-humiliation factor is still putting a damper on your enthusiasm for trying a class, here are some guidelines that will help ease you in, stumble-free:

✔ Do one component of a move at a time. For example, during an aerobic dance or kickboxing class, you might have a combination that incorporates a lower body move (a jump or a kick) with an upper body move (a biceps curl or a punch). Try the leg movement first. When you feel comfortable with the foot pattern, then, and only then, add the arm movement.

✔ Skip the cartwheels and other tricky steps. Some fitness classes — especially step — are very complicated. (Here's an insider secret: In many cases, when a routine becomes highly complicated, in order to perform the moves, the intensity must come down. So a complex class doesn't always give you the best calorie-burning workout. A simple class that lets you focus on getting your heart rate up and working your muscles thoroughly instead of memorizing lots of complex moves is often the better workout.) But that doesn't mean you have to leave the class if you can't follow the routine exactly. Modify the moves. A good instructor should always show easier versions of her routine. For example, instead of doing a turn, kick, jump, and fancy arm pattern, you can alternate jogging and marching in place. Instead of flying around your step, you can stick to the basic steps where you step up and down repeatedly or alternate knee lifts.

✔ Perform an easier version of an exercise if you feel out of breath or if your body hurts. Not every exercise or movement will be right for you, and on different days you may feel more or less energetic. Listen to your body and do what feels best for you; don't feel like you have to do everything the teacher does. A good teacher should encourage you to stop or modify your movements. If you get a dirty look because you're doing something different from the rest of the class (and we've heard horror stories of some instructors bullying their students), stay away from that teacher.

✔ If you can't follow a complicated routine, don't take it out on yourself. One sign of a poor teacher is the inability to break down choreography and repeat it often enough so that students can follow. You shouldn't have to take a teacher's class for a month before you can follow the steps. You should be able to do it the first time. Keep taking different classes until you find an instructor that teaches in the style that you can follow.

✔ If you move in the wrong direction, or do something different than the rest of the class, relax. The others are probably staring at themselves in the mirror, not you.

If you're choreography-phobic, stay away from step classes unless they are billed as being for beginners. (Step is the workout where you step up and down off an 8-12-inch bench. You can step on it in different directions and with different arm and foot patterns.) The problem is, some instructors have turned this great calorie-blasting workout into a Broadway dance class on a bench. That's fine if you're familiar with the step moves and want a brain challenge during your workout, but if you're just looking for a fun, simple way to sweat, you might want to try an easier-to-follow class.

Tough guy takes a dance class

After years of playing football and spending his practice sessions doing athletic drills and weight lifting, Tony decided to give jazz dance classes a try. Although he expected to excel like he always had in physical activities, he stumbled through a few twists and twirls and walked out humiliated. It was tougher than he'd ever imagined. But he stuck to it, and after just a few classes, he found his coordination, body control, and balance improving. Fitness is specific, so no matter how fit you are, when you try something new, there will always be a learning curve to overcome. The good news is, the fitter you are, the easier your body will adapt to new styles of movement.

Group Fitness Classes

We outline the general types of group fitness classes that you'll find offered at a health club near you. We give you a basic description about each class, but remember that teachers vary, so while one aerobic-dance class might have all-cardio movements, another might mix some aerobic-dance moves, some step moves, some kickboxing moves, and weight work. Check the following chart to see the general fitness emphasis for each type of class. Keep in mind, however, that it's hard to generalize about the benefits that you can get from each type of class because it all depends upon the specific exercises that are used and the way that they are taught. A circuit-training class, for example, may give you a good cardio workout, especially if it incorporates lots of aerobic intervals such as step-ups and jumping jacks. An aerobics class may include a good deal of stretching and sculpting moves that can enhance your flexibility and strength.

Aerobics (multi-impact)

You can wiggle, jiggle, and jump to your heart's content in this traditional aerobics class. Aerobics started out as being mostly high-impact (that is, you performed most of the moves with jumping and jogging variations). It then evolved into a nonjump format called *low-impact* (see the following section). Typical moves are stepping side to side and marching in place. To keep the joy of the jump into the mix, multi-impact classes were born, interspersing high- and low-impact moves. Multi-impact aerobics is a cardio stamina and muscular endurance class with a variety of leg and arm patterns, jumps, and moves on the floor. Sample moves include jumping jacks, kicks, knee lifts, punches, biceps curls, marching in place, and so on.

Some movement combinations have you jog or kick while punching or pushing your arms up. Raising your arms over your head can raise the intensity slightly. If you're out of breath, lower your arms. Also, you can always modify the jumping moves with a low-impact version (marching instead of jogging, for example).

Aerobics (low-impact)

If you like to shuffle and hustle, this is the workout for you. Low-impact aerobics is a cardio stamina and muscular endurance class that includes stationary and traveling patterns on the floor coupled with a variety of arm movements. Sample moves include stepping side to side, low kicking, lunging, and marching. The class has less pounding than multi-impact aerobics, but that doesn't mean it's easier. Usually you move across the floor in different directions at a fast pace in order to keep your heart rate up.

A *grapevine* is a classic aerobic dance move that you'll find in nearly every class. Two side steps to the right and then to the left (or four single footsteps each way) comprise this move. In a regular standing position, step your right foot to the side. Now cross your left foot behind the right. Step your right foot to the right again, and then bring your left foot together with your right. Think right, left, right, together. Now for the other side: step left, right, left, together. The second step crosses in front of or behind the first foot that steps out for a smoother progression. See, it's easier than it sounds. Take it slow at first, and you won't trip over your own feet!

Funk aerobics

If fitness with attitude is your thang, you'll love the coolness quotient you get from funky classes. Expect to feel like you're auditioning for an MTV dance video. Funk aerobics is a low-impact aerobics class filled with hip hop and dance-style moves. The music is usually slower so you get a heavy beat. One caveat: These classes can be complicated. Some fabulous teachers out there can break down Janet Jackson-style combinations so well that you slip right into them never knowing you were capable of moving in such a way. Then there are other teachers who may look good themselves doing the steps, but leave their students flailing unfunkily behind. Still, even mastering one teeny dance step can be fun.

To make the klutz in you feel a little bit funky, identify the different components of each move and master each separately before trying to do them all at once. First, feel the beat of the music. It's usually heavier and the emphasis is on the down beat. Move your head or your hips to match this rhythm. Experiment with changing the speed and length of your footsteps. Funkier moves are usually shorter and choppier than the same move performed in an unfunky way.

Step aerobics

Six words: *it used to be so simple.* Step aerobics is a low-impact aerobics class performed while stepping on and off a 4-10-inch platform. It started in the 1980s as an easy-to-follow workout. In fact, in the early days, it was one of the first fitness classes that appealed to men: There were no cutesy dance moves. All you had to do was step up and down, and boy, did you work up a sweat! Then, the step instructors started getting tired of doing the same old thing. Their creative juices ran rampant and they made the choreography so complex that in classes today you'll find people hopping around all four sides of the step, twisting and turning backwards and forwards, all the while throwing in arm moves, high kicks, knee lifts, and grapevines.

Step instructors even use a special vocabulary associated with step: *over-the-top, turn step, repeater, indecision move,* and so on. It's not only extremely difficult but downright impossible for a newcomer to pick up the moves. The problem is, as the classes have gotten trickier, the music has been speeded up (increasing the tripability factor). Plus, some of the turning moves can be risky on the knees.

Fortunately, many instructors are realizing that this potentially great workout may peter out if new members aren't able to do it, or if the injury risk increases, so some classes are going back to the basics and keeping the highly choreographic moves for the advanced classes only.

If you're in a class with lots of twists and turns on the step, don't bother to try to follow. These moves can be extremely stressful to the knees. You're better off doing the basic step movements and keeping your heart rate up, rather than trying to follow complicated foot patterns.

Cross-training class

Variety is the buzzword in this class. You'll usually incorporate lots of different types of both cardio and strength moves within one high-energy session. Often instructors offer this class outside, and you use nature as your fitness tools: You climb up steps, run up hills, and do athletic drills on the ground (all with a series of push-ups, jumping jacks, and other basic calisthenic exercises thrown in). Some indoor classes have backtracked and taken the school recess approach, using hula hoops, balls, mini-trampolines, and jump ropes.

These classes are usually easy to follow, fun to do, and great for beginners.

Circuit training

A high-energy mix of easy-to-follow cardio and strength exercises make this interval-style workout quite tough. Different variations of the class include an all-weight-machine circuit where you move from machine to machine and a boot-camp-style session where you do a variety of push-ups, weight moves, and jumping jacks.

This class is usually filled with participants with red faces. That's because the quick pace and tough moves can push the intensity level very high. Take it easy if you're just starting out.

Martial arts–based aerobics

Believe it or not, Tae Bo was not the first workout of its kind. Martial arts-based aerobics have been around for about ten years. The famous infomercial that shows jabs, hooks, and roundhouse kicks sparked the interest of the masses. The irony is that Tae Bo-esque style classes are very similar to multi-impact aerobics classes. The beauty of this style class is that it's easy to follow.

Basically, all you do is punch, kick, jog, and jump. The movements are repetitive and simple (step instructors take note), and the workout has a high sweat value. Spin-off variations, however, depend upon whether the style uses karate, boxing, or kickboxing-based moves. Depending on the teacher, some classes are very athletic, and other classes combine aerobic choreography with the moves for a more fluid routine. Some of these classes also use punching bags to up the ante.

In your excitement over how tough you feel in these classes, it's easy to punch and kick too hard. Avoid jarring your joints by controlling the stopping phase each time you extend your arm or leg. Try not to kick higher than your flexibility allows — executing a swift, high kick with force is not the time to sneak your stretching in! Most guidelines advise that you kick at around knee-to-hip level.

Bodysculpting

Sculpt is the word that superceded the girly 1980s term *tone* back when women wanted to be firm but were afraid of their muscles. Bodysculpting is a nonaerobic strength training class that uses dumbbells, barbells, and sometimes rubber resistance bands. Check your coordination skills at the door; you won't need them here. Most classes do one to three sets of a variety of exercises (like those that are in Part IV) to work your major muscle groups. Different teachers have different techniques — some move faster, some move slower.

Bodysculpting is a good way to weight train if you're not motivated enough to drag your butt to the gym and weight train on your own, or if you are a beginner and feel unsure of what to do on your own in a weight room at the gym.

Select several pairs of weights to use throughout the class. Since different muscles are stronger than others, you'll want to switch depending upon the exercise you do.

BodyPump

"Pump that Body" must have been the song that inspired the name of this branded, pre-choreographed weights class. BodyPump is a nonaerobic, strength training class similar to a regular bodysculpting class except that it uses barbells instead of dumbbells. The instructors also follow certain set routines, so you'll find different classes at different places all following a similar format. The moves are all basic moves like squats and biceps curls done at a slow-to-moderate pace. This class tends to focus on building muscular endurance, so expect lots of repetitions.

Some moves may be difficult to do with a heavy barbell. Don't be afraid to move slower than the rest of the class if it feels more comfortable for your body.

Pilates

Pilates (pronounced *puh-la-tees*) or Pilates-based classes are a nonaerobic, basic body conditioning workout that uses weights and rubber resistance tools, as well as spring-resistance machines, to target the major muscle groups. Usually these classes don't use music. Based in dance, Pilates uses some unusual movement patterns and also emphasizes flexibility.

These moves are done slowly, but since they were originally designed to be done by dancers who are used to extreme positions, some of them can be stressful on the knees, back, and shoulders. If something feels uncomfortable, don't do it.

Yoga

Yoga is an age-old practice that has been popularized to become a stretch and conditioning workout. Different forms of yoga emphasize different aspects of the technique such as breathing, meditation, body positions, and so on. However, most purists don't view yoga as an exercise method but as a path to spiritual enlightenment and personal achievement.

All forms of yoga base themselves on a set number of basic yoga postures known as *asanas*. Some of these postures may require excessive levels of flexibility in order to hold the position. For most people, overstretching joint tissues to the extreme causes a loss in joint stability. Yoga is great for increasing suppleness, balance, and flexibility, but beware of pushing too far.

The resurgence in interest in yoga has brought an awareness of balance back to many exercisers' lives. Key benefits you'll get from yoga include deep breathing, enhanced mental focus, and improved balance.

Indoor cycling

Who would have ever thought that riding a stationary bike could be so exciting? Indoor cycling is a group class on a stationary bike and one of the hottest classes in health clubs right now. One of the most well known classes is Spinning. Meant to simulate an outdoor cycle ride inside, these classes are tough. An instructor on a bike plays a variety of music and talks you through your paces. You might pretend to climb a big hill and then speed down it, all the while envisioning your fellow indoor cyclists racing alongside of you. You'll get a great cardio stamina workout and develop muscular endurance in your lower body.

Many classes push participants to the extreme. Two practices in many classes are counterproductive: spinning the wheels too fast, or pedaling at a high number of revolutions per minute (rpm) with little resistance, and jumping, lifting on and off the seat from a sitting to a standing position repeatedly. Both of these techniques feel difficult and have the perception of being advanced movements. However, they don't actually make you work harder or burn many more calories, and they can be extremely stressful on the knees. Your best bet is to stay mostly seated and cycle with enough resistance that your rpm is within the 60-90 range.

Stomp

Just when the stair machine started to get boring, someone decided to follow the lead of indoor cycling and create a choreographed set of moves to do in a group. Stomp is an instructor-led, group-machine class performed on the Stairmaster. Participants switch intensity and mimic different types of climbs.

Machines can get boring, so any type of external motivation or technique variation can be a good change. Watch out, though, for moves that may stress your back and knees. Always listen to your body.

Trekking

Tired of watching the seconds go by? Trekking is an instructor-led, group treadmill workout. This class is great if you've been stuck doing the same old walk or jog on a treadmill and need some impetus to stick to it. The instructor leads you through different speeds and levels of incline. The treadmill is one of the best machines around. Whether you walk it or run it, you're sure to get a great workout in this class.

Don't be afraid to run if you're a walker or to try fast walking if you're a runner. In this type of class you can experiment with smaller doses of an activity that you're not sure is right for you.

Crew class

Crew class is an instructor-led, group rowing class on Concept II ergometers. You are led through different intensity levels and speeds and may simulate racing on a scull or rowboat.

Rowing technique involves perfectly timed coordination between your upper body and lower body. The movement can be tricky to master so instruction is always a good thing.

Chapter 24

Strutting Your Stuff on the Field

● ●

In This Chapter

▶ Cross-training for team sports

▶ Tips to enhance performance

● ●

Sports are about more than just exercise. A certain ambience transcends the exercise — the focus on the immediate moment at hand, the stillness before the next big move is made, the unity between players (even those on the opposite team), plus the exhilaration (and defeat) you feel when you catch (or miss) a ball thrown or kicked your way. Something about sports brings us back to our prehistoric roots. Then it was about the hunt for food and water, now it's the pursuit of a common goal in the game.

Since team sports are competitive, they carry more risk than gym-style exercise. Unexpected twists, turns, and charging opponents are factors you can only prepare for but never control. Sports are generally more skill-based than fitness-based, although to do well you need to be fit to last longer and produce the requisite power to execute the skills well.

Sports are a great antidote for those who hate to exercise, because you're not just running to nowhere on a machine, you're running after something or away from someone. But it's important to start playing at lower intensities and get fit enough to play the sport before you go for the gold and try to perform heroic game-saving moves. To lower your intensity with activities such as jogging and cycling, you just need to slow down. With a fast sport, that's not always possible without pulling yourself out of the game. One way to lower the intensity during super-fast activities like basketball is to play with players who are your own skill level, rather than those who are so much better than you. That way, you won't be gasping to keep up.

Sports help develop hand/eye coordination and other skills and reflexes. Most fast sports involve some degree of power or explosive moves. If you're training at a competitive level and are fit enough to do so, adding plyometric training may help improve your game. Most sports also involve moving in many directions and planes of motion. Agility drills like the ones we suggest in Chapter 21 are excellent preparation. Because each sport has its own unique movement patterns (swinging a bat, jumping and making a basket, serving a tennis ball, and so on), to improve your ability to do these tasks, you must train in ways that specifically mimic that movement. This can be done through repetition of the actions themselves and by doing strength movements that follow the same patterns or target the same muscle groups.

We put together a rundown on the seven top sports that you're most likely to play. Check out the chart below to see which areas of fitness you'll improve by playing. As you can see, most sports are cross-training regimens unto themselves since they develop many components of fitness. But again, it's hard to generalize because what you get out of these activities depends upon how you play. You might get a tremendous cardio workout from playing tennis if all you do is chase the balls that you miss! But if you have a killer tennis serve that your opponent can never return, you might stand still for an hour with your right arm being the only thing getting a workout.

For each of the following sports, we outline key things you should know, including a few recommended stretches and strength moves found in Part IV or described individually that may help improve your performance in that sport. For a more comprehensive study of everything you need to know about your favorite sport, there's a ...For Dummies book to guide you along, so check out the titles at your local bookstore.

Basketball

If you're bored with exercise, basketball is a great game to pick up. Since it moves so quickly, you don't have time to think about anything else. If you've never played, it's a good idea to develop a base level of fitness first and practice the basic drills before plunging your body into a head-to-head game with seasoned players. The drills can be just as fun and just as good for exercise as the game.

Basketball focuses on cardio stamina, muscular endurance, power, agility, balance, speed, and dynamic flexibility.

Pros and Cons

As a fun, fast game that will get you in great shape, basketball burns lots of calories and is convenient to participate in as most suburban driveways, parks, schools, YMCAs, sports clubs, and gyms have hoops. Public facilities often have round-the-clock games in progress, so you can squeeze into a pickup game with others. Bonus: If you play with short people, you don't need to be tall. You can vary the game by playing with one to six players on the court at a time.

If you play with those who are better than you, you're more likely to push your-self too hard. Also, it's a tough game with lots of jumping, side-to-side move-ments, and quick changes, making it easy to twist ankles and so on. When everyone's up close and scrambling for the ball, elbows fly around — the last thing anyone worries about is hitting your nose, so watch out for yours.

What you need to know

Make sure to wear basketball shoes for maximum ankle stability.

To do well in basketball, you need body awareness and the ability to control how you move. Dance, aerobics, and yoga can help target your coordination, balance, agility, and dynamic control. Being especially conscious of lifting weights with precision translates into moving with speed and grace on the court.

Recommended training, cross-training, and stretches

During the season, improve your performance by including the following in your training sessions: agility drills, jump training (including plyometrics if you're fit enough), leg strength exercises, core body strength, and upper body endurance work, such as aerobics, dribbling, shooting, and passing drills.

During the off-season, you can ensure that your workouts stay balanced by cross-training with swimming, rowing, and cycling.

You should always warm up and stretch all major muscles, but be sure to spend a little extra time on the following muscle groups that can get over-worked in this game. Check out Chapters 15 and 28 for exercises to loosen up your hamstrings, torso, gluteals, quads, calves, soleus, and chest.

To enhance your basketball performance, include these exercises in your training plan:

✔ Squat presses (see Chapter 18)

✔ Jump lunges (see Chapter 20; you should be in good condition before attempting this power move)

✔ Lateral hops (see Chapter 20; you should be in good condition before trying this power move)

Softball and Baseball

For many Americans, baseball and softball bring back the warm fuzzies from childhood. Remember those evenings when you'd play catch with your dad right before supper? Or how about those pickup games the neighborhood kids would throw together immediately after school? Something about throwing and catching just feels good. So even if you don't have a team to play with, grab a friend, two gloves, and ball and go play catch. It's great exercise — especially if you're a little rusty and have to chase the ball.

Softball and baseball build strength and flexibility. Depending on the position you play, and whether you're playing slow-pitch softball or baseball or fast-pitch softball, you'll hone different areas of fitness. You can develop hand-eye coordination from throwing, catching, and hitting, and you can improve your reaction reflexes by responding to quickly moving balls.

Pros and cons

Softball and baseball are fun. City and company leagues nationwide offer both slow-pitch and fast-pitch games. When you hit the ball in what is known as the *sweet spot,* smack in the thickest part of the bat with a perfect swing, there's no better feeling.

Would it be un-American to suggest that baseball or softball has any downsides? Although we don't want to put this sport down, we must tell you that for starters, you need equipment: a glove, a ball, and cleats for the field. You need skill, but as long as you start at an easy level, such as slow-pitch softball, you'll improve by playing.

What you need to know

Throwing can be stressful to the shoulder, especially if you try to throw too hard or too far. Always warm up your shoulders for at least ten minutes before throwing. Do shoulder circles forward and backward, and move your arms up and down and in and out in all different directions. Always start with soft, easy throws. Gradually increase the distance and speed.

If you're a novice, just remember one thing: When the ball is coming toward you, keep your eye on the ball and block it with your glove. You'll never get hurt that way. Martica learned this the hard way. During her high school years as a fast-pitch pitcher she trained to dodge or stop infield hits. Then during one game, her reflexes were a second too slow — the batter hit a line-drive straight into her eye. Ouch!

Recommended training, cross-training, and stretches

During the season, improve your performance by including the following in your training sessions: sprint drills, agility drills, strength training, flexibility, throwing, catching, and hitting.

During the off-season, you can ensure that your workouts stay balanced by cross-training with running, basketball, and tennis.

You should always warm up and stretch all major muscles, but be sure to spend a little extra time on the following muscle groups that can get overworked in this sport. Check out Chapters 15 and 28 for exercises to loosen up your chest, hamstrings, quadriceps, gluteals, and triceps.

Get your body primed for action by including these moves in your training sessions:

 ✔ Squats (see Chapter 16)

 ✔ Military presses overhead (see Chapter 17)

 ✔ Lat pulldowns (see Chapter 19)

 ✔ Ab twists on ball (see Chapter 17)

 ✔ Back extensions (see Chapter 17)

Soccer

Soccer is a quiet giant in the United States. Although it's been a popular sport for high school and college participants for many years, on a professional level it doesn't receive the media coverage that football, basketball, and baseball do. This is changing, though. The Women's World Cup Championships in 1999, starring the U.S. women's team, brought in some of the highest ratings ever for a televised sport. It's *the* chosen sport of the rest of the world. If you show up to a big city park, you're likely to meet a lot of new foreign friends. Soccer is a great workout as it's essentially a 90-minute group run with quick action to move the ball toward the goal.

Be prepared to really work hard while playing this sport. Your cardio stamina, speed, muscular endurance, leg strength, balance, and agility benefit from soccer.

Pros and cons

You'll get in great cardio shape fast playing this, but if you're not familiar with the positions, you need to learn them. For just like football, every player has a different task. Soccer is an easy game to learn but requires a lot of skill. Watch out for other feet trying to trip you up — a recipe for falls.

What you need to know

Unlike most other sports, you can use your head but not your hands. You'll need to include sprint and agility drills in your practice sessions to prepare for the fast-flying kicks you'll encounter from the opposite side.

Recommended training, cross-training, and stretches

During the season, improve your performance by including running, sprint drills, agility drills, and lower body strength work in your training sessions.

During the off-season, you can ensure that your workouts stay balanced by cross-training with upper body strength training and swimming.

You should always warm up and stretch all major muscles, but be sure to spend a little extra time on the following muscle groups that can get over-worked in this game. Check out Chapters 15 and 28 for exercises to loosen up your quadriceps, hamstrings, gluteals, adductors, calves, soleus, and lower back before and after playing.

Wow them with your speed and nimbleness by including these moves in your training sessions:

- Jump lunges (see Chapter 20)
- Agility drills (see Chapter 21)
- Lunge scissor kicks (see Chapter 18)

Football

Football brings out the aggression in players. So even if you're playing flag football, be careful; every bone has the potential to be injured. Football is a great team sport, and chances are, if you're a guy, you have lots of willing friends to play with you. If you're a woman, you might have to earn their respect to join in. Flag and touch football offer an alternative to the harder-hitting tackle football and rugby.

Different positions require different strengths. Overall, football players need upper and lower body strength, flexibility, agility, power, and cardio stamina.

Pros and cons

Football is an easy game to pick up in the park and a great weekend past-time. Even throwing the football back and forth is good exercise. Unfortunately, the rules and plays can get complicated. Every position requires different skills.

What you need to know

Injuries most often occur in the fourth quarter when players lose their energy. Stamina and muscle-lasting power are crucial, not only to keep your energy levels up, but to muster up the last bit of energy needed to make the final touchdown.

Things get knocked around, so wear a mouthpiece (buy one at the drugstore) and as much padding as you can. Even if you're a weekend football player, a pair of padded bike shorts can't hurt.

Recommended training, cross-training, and stretches

During the season, improve your performance by including running, interval sprints, weight lifting for the upper and lower body, and plyometrics or power moves (if you're fit enough) in your training sessions.

During the off-season, you can ensure that your workouts stay balanced by cross-training with basketball, soccer, swimming, dance, aerobics, and cycling.

You should always warm up and stretch all major muscles, but be sure to spend a little extra time on the following muscle groups that can get over-worked in this game. Check out Chapters 15 and 28 for exercises to loosen up your gluteals, quadriceps, hamstrings, torso, and lats before getting started.

To help prevent fourth-quarter injuries, incorporate these exercises into your training plan:

- Dynamic side lunges (see Chapter 18)
- Squats (see Chapter 16)
- Bentover deltoids (see Chapter 17)
- Military presses overhead (see Chapter 17)
- Agility drills (see Chapter 21)

Tony developed his own brand of football when he was a kid. He and his brother played slo-mo football in the living room. The confined space and body control required to play indoors ended up being a good workout.

Volleyball

Volleyball became cool in the 1990s when the lithe, muscular bodies of beach volleyball players like Gabrielle Reese became a regular part of ESPN. You can join in on pickup volleyball games everywhere from the beaches of California to the sand courts of Central Park in New York City. City leagues nationwide offer year-round opportunities to play. Volleyball is a fun game that is as tough as you make it. It's perfect for novice players at the park, but it can become very competitive, too. Variations of the sport include playing on the beach or playing on a court with one to six players per side. You'll develop strength, cardio stamina, flexibility, power, and agility from playing this game.

Pros and cons

You can play this easy game indoors or outdoors. The fewer the people playing, the more challenging the game becomes. Volleyball has enough consistent movement to chalk up a good calorie burn. This is a real team game, as the constant communication on how to play the ball must be shared continuously between teammates.

The only cons are that you need a net and a court. Plus, say goodbye to long fingernails; the direct hand contact you make with the ball on serves and volleys means they'll stay short.

What you need to know

Beginners like to bump the ball by making a fist with both hands and whamming it as far as they can. This is a sure sign that the ball will go out of the court and that you don't know how to play volleyball. To bump properly, you need to place your forearms side-by-side and lightly clasp one hand on top of the other. Your palms and inner forearms should face up. Keep the elbows close and capture the ball from underneath, moving it with control by using some arm movement but mostly propulsion from your springing body.

Recommended training, cross-training, and stretches

During the season, improve your performance by including the following in your training sessions: Jump training, running, sprint training, aerobics, and upper body strength work.

During the off-season, you can ensure that your workouts stay balanced by cross-training with swimming, cycling, and basketball.

You should always warm up and stretch all major muscles, but be sure to spend a little extra time on the following muscle groups that can get overworked in this sport. Check out Chapters 15 and 28 for exercises to loosen up your triceps, lats, gluteals, and back.

Power up your abilities by including these exercises in your training sessions:

- ✔ Slalom jump twists (see Chapter 20)
- ✔ Jump lunges (see Chapter 20)
- ✔ Agility drills (see Chapter 21)

Golf

Golf is not just a game; it's a lifestyle because it's one of the most addictive sports around. It doesn't just appeal to the older, country club crowd anymore, and plaid pants aren't required. Golfers like Tiger Woods have brought a new spirit to the game that tests your skill, control, balance, and flexibility. Providing you go cartless, you can also get a good cardio walk over the course of an 18-hole game. A new spin-off, called speed-golf, factors the amount of time it takes you to play the course, as well as the number of shots you make, into your score.

Pros and cons

The mental component of determining which club to use to hit the ball and how to approach each stroke on the course is a fulfilling challenge. However, to get into the game you need lessons, equipment, and access to a golf course (which isn't always easy). If you also opt for the Mr. Rogers-style sweaters and two-toned shoes, golf can be quite an investment.

What you need to know

It takes time to become a good golfer, which is why the game is a lifelong sport that you can play well into your old age.

Power in your swing is dependent on both flexibility in your torso, stability, control of the movement, and good technique. The twisting action of a swing can aggravate back problems, so make sure to include lots of core body strength work in your training routine.

Recommended training, cross-training, and stretches

During the season, improve your performance by adding walking, strength work, and stretching in your training sessions. You should also practice your swing.

During the off-season, you can ensure that your workouts stay balanced by cross-training with swimming, aerobics, and cycling.

You should always warm up and stretch all major muscles, but be sure to spend a little extra time on the following muscle groups that can get overworked in this game. Check out Chapters 15 and 28 for exercises to loosen up your torso, hamstrings, and back.

Maximize your performance by including these exercises into your training plan:

- Lateral raises (see Chapter 17)
- Military presses overhead (see Chapter 17)
- Triceps kickbacks (see Chapter 17)
- Lat pulldowns (see Chapter 19)

Racket Sports

Whacking something with a racket is so much fun that lots of ways to do it have evolved. You can choose from tennis, squash, racquetball, badminton, Ping-Pong, and paddle ball. Each of these works different aspects of fitness, but you can expect to build cardio stamina, muscular endurance and strength, and coordination.

Pros and cons

Racket sports are fun to play, and you can play all your life. Once you're good and you're playing with someone of an equivalent level, you can get a good cardio workout. However, twists and turns can lead to ankle sprains and other injuries. Play with someone of your own level to ensure that you don't overexert yourself.

What you need to know

Take lessons to learn how to serve and return properly. Good technique prevents shoulder and elbow injuries later. In faster games, such as squash and racquetball, wear eye goggles for protection.

To build up strength in the shoulder joint, include exercises for your rotator cuff muscles in your training plan. Holding a light weight, bend your elbow into a biceps curl, keeping your elbow bent 90 degrees and pressed to your rib cage. Slowly move your hand towards your chest to rotate your shoulder inward, and then out to the side, held away from your body to rotate the shoulder outward. Repeat 8-12 times, three days a week.

Recommended training, cross-training, and stretches

During the season, improve your performance by adding agility drills, upper and lower body strength work, aerobics, and core strength work in your training sessions.

During the off-season, you can ensure that your workouts stay balanced by cross-training with swimming, cycling, and flexibility exercises.

You should always warm up and stretch all major muscles, but be sure to spend a little extra time on the following muscle groups that can get overworked in this game. Check out Chapters 15 and 28 for exercises to loosen up your triceps, biceps, chest, hamstrings, quadriceps, and calves.

Fire up your court-side moves by including these exercises into your training sessions:

- Agility drills (see Chapter 21)
- Triceps kickbacks (see Chapter 17)
- Lateral raises (see Chapter 17)
- Back lunges (see Chapter 16)
- Side lunges (see Chapter 18)
- Biceps curls (see Chapter 17)

Part VI
The Part of Tens

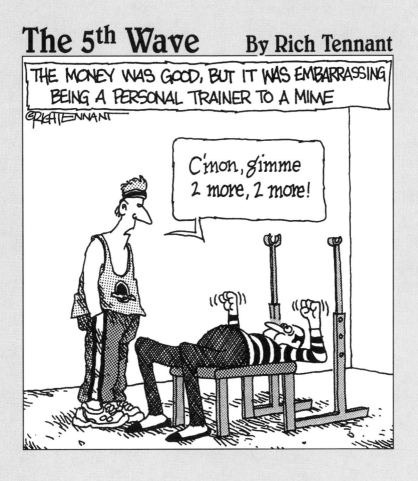

The 5th Wave   By Rich Tennant

THE MONEY WAS GOOD, BUT IT WAS EMBARRASSING BEING A PERSONAL TRAINER TO A MIME

C'mon, gimme 2 more, 2 more!

In this part . . .

We present the top ten things you should know about muscles, ten ways to maximize your rest days (do any of these have to do with a trip to the Bahamas?), ten ways to stick to your new program (is snorkeling in the Bahamas included?), and ten great bench stretches (which also can be done from your beach chair).

Chapter 25

Ten Things You Should Know about Muscles

In This Chapter

▶ Burning calories with weights

▶ Toning your body to change its shape

▶ Building friendships with your aging muscles

Muscles used to be something that only bodybuilders, wimps on the beach, and athletes worried about. No longer. Research shows that muscle is the aging body's best friend because we lose muscle as we become more sedentary over the years. Once your muscles diminish, your posture, firm body parts, stability, agility, strength, power, and good looks go downhill as well. In this chapter, we wow you with some interesting info about muscles. We also clear up some misleading assumptions that people have made over the years.

Weights Rev Your Engine

Most people go cardio-mad when they're trying to burn calories. Although weight training doesn't burn as many calories as, say, running, in a single session, the muscle mass you salvage can account for an 8 percent increase in your overall metabolism over the long term. So, depending upon your height and weight, that increase in your metabolism can equate to about 200-300 extra calories a day that your body burns when it has more muscle mass. It's like diet-free dieting. Over time, that 200 extra calories a day that your body is using can help you lose weight! That's one reason why men and athletes can seem to eat more without gaining weight.

You Can't Get Toned without Getting Strong

Many women shy away from heavier weights because they fear looking like Arnold Schwarzenegger. They want to look *toned,* so they pick the lightest, least scary-looking dumbbell possible. (Heaven forbid if they were to get big and strong; they just want *tone* or firmness.) Tone is thought to be a more attractive, female-friendly look. But tone is simply a characteristic of a strong muscle, so if you're not trying to get strong, you're not going to get very toned or firm. The irony is that a handbag (that you've stuffed with everything but the kitchen sink), grocery bag (filled with high fiber like fruits, beans, and vegetables), or laundry basket (after avoiding the laundromat for a week) are heavier than the kind of weight most women lift on a regular basis, so a workout using light weights may be less challenging than what they are capable of doing. The stimulus simply won't be enough to do anything to the muscle but develop more endurance.

To get firm, a muscle must get strong. The only way to increase strength is to get your muscle to exert more force than it normally does. It will adapt to the challenge by getting stronger. Even if a woman is lifting extremely heavy weights, her lower testosterone levels make it almost impossible to develop an excessive amount of muscle mass.

Two-Pound Dumbbells Won't Cut It

If you're trying to improve your muscle strength and you're lifting very light weights, you're not going to see much improvement. To develop strength, you need to work a muscle to fatigue within 30 to 90 seconds. Most people can accomplish this when they lift enough weight so that the muscle is fatigued after doing about 8-12 repetitions of an exercise or roughly using about 75 percent of the maximum force a muscle can exert. A weight that's too light may take minutes and hundreds of repetitions to fatigue — so the effect is improved endurance, not strength. If you want to be firm, you've got to be strong.

Weights Can Reshape

If any kind of exercise can improve what you were born with, weights can — to a certain degree, anyway. We're born with a predetermined distribution of fat cells and muscle-fiber type. (Refresh yourself on muscles and metabolism in Part II.) A regular program of strength training can shift your proportion of fat to muscle, causing you to feel firmer and look leaner. Plus, building curvier body parts can rebalance an unproportioned body.

Weights and Cardio Don't Mix

You've seen the power walkers and even runners in the park lugging around small hand weights or working up a sweat with ankle weights slowing them down. You might have even seen the occasional step or aerobics class where light weights are swung around during the fast cardio moves. Grabbing a pair of light weights and pumping your arms like a wild person during a cardio workout isn't as effective as you might think. Studies show that using one- or two-pound weights doesn't increase the intensity of your workout. If you burn any more calories at all from doing this, it amounts to an additional 10 to 20 calories over an hour-long session, which is hardly worth the effort since simply picking up your pace without weights can boost the energy expenditure by up to 50 percent.

Plus, you exacerbate the stress on your joints when the weights are swung back and forth with momentum. In order to protect your body parts, it's a good idea to slow down, which burns even fewer calories and defeats the whole purpose of picking up the weights in the first place! And you won't get stronger using weights this light. Your best bet is to leave the weights on the rack and pick up your intensity by speeding up and working harder.

Women Are as Strong as Men

Well, sort of. Studies show that the average man can lift about 50 percent more weight than the average woman. However, this is only because, pound for pound, they have more muscle and less fat per square inch of skin. When these variables are accounted for and a comparison of strength versus muscle mass is done, women are equally strong.

It Ain't Easy Being Big and Bulky

So you *want* to get big and build muscles that you can be proud of? On the few forays you've made into the weight room, you've probably found that building bulk is not as easy as just pumping iron a couple of days a week. Even bodybuilders find it difficult to increase their muscle size. (That's why they spend hours in the gyms lifting weights that weigh more than most people. Plus they often take hormones to help out.) The fact is less than 1 percent of the population has the genetic or hormonal predisposition to build big muscle. Women with minimal testosterone levels have a nearly impossible chance. Plus, the taller you are, the less bulky you'll look because longer limbs have longer muscles.

You can develop more muscle mass, but remember that it takes at least 12 weeks to see any increases in the hypertrophy, or size of muscle. Plus, you're not going to look very defined if you have excess body fat. You can get sculpted, admirable curves, but it takes time and dedication. Concentrate on overloading your muscles with heavier weights gradually and including regular cardio workouts in your routine.

A Flabby Future

Maturity may come with age, but strength doesn't. As you age, you can lose five to six pounds of muscle per decade. If you've been dieting for years with massive weight fluctuations, you can lose even more. Because muscle cells require energy to exist in your body, the more muscle fiber you have, the more energy your body requires. (Translation: You have a higher metabolism, which means you can eat more without gaining weight. Sounds good to us!) The downside is that losing muscle mass (as the result of becoming a couch potato) slows down your metabolism, making it much easier to gain unwelcome pounds. You can prevent it all by lifting weights regularly.

Muscles Need to Rest

When you lift weights, you push the muscle fibers to work just a teensy bit too hard. They get so tired that they need some time to repair. On their time off, they like to relax, build themselves back up, and get stronger. (We believe that relaxing is best done on a Caribbean island, or at the very least, on comp days off work, sleeping in late.) For best results, you should wait approximately 48 hours in between sessions and lift two or three times per week. If you're on a heavy-duty program of switching the muscles you work and training every day, your rest days will be those that aren't spent training a particular muscle group.

Weights Protect Weak Joints

If you have back problems, knee pain, arthritis, bursitis, or other joint weaknesses, in most cases, weight training can help alleviate stress on the joints by making the surrounding muscles stronger. It may feel uncomfortable, or even painful, to exercise with these conditions, but sometimes *not* exercising will cause the muscles to atrophy (get weaker), making the problem even worse. ***Remember:*** Always check with your doctor first before undertaking any exercise program.

Chapter 26

Ten Ways to Maximize Rest Days

In This Chapter

▶ Stretching for relaxation

▶ Breathing deeply

▶ Dancing out your stress

*Y*ou've been running and jumping and pushing and pulling. You've bathed in a pool of glorious sweat. Now you deserve a day of cross-training glory. This is it: your rest day. So what are you going to do with it? Sure, you can rest, but we have some even better suggestions. You can relax your mind and body, from head to toe. We've picked some great ways to release the tension of over-worked muscles and help you forget about the stresses of your everyday life.

Stretch Away Stress

Although we've only recommended that you stretch three days a week in the Cross-Training Plans, unless you've been doing extreme yoga for 20 years or you've got the elasticity of Gumby, it never hurts to stretch a little more. You might be stiffer-than-usual if you're stressed out, because you might be sub-consciously tightening muscles in your body. Do these quick tension-busters:

✔ Lie on your back and hug your knees into your chest. Keep your head on the ground and gently rock your body from side to side.

✔ Still lying down, rest your body in the center, and then slowly circle your shoulders forward. Make the circles big, bringing the shoulders up toward the ceiling and then down toward your hips. Then circle your shoulder blades toward the floor and then back up toward your ears. Feel any tight spots in the shoulders and roll them out. Then reverse directions.

✔ Relax your shoulders. Keeping your head on the ground, slowly roll your head from side to side. Press the back of your neck into the ground to give yourself a head massage as you rotate the neck.

> ✔ Relax your head, and then reach both arms over your head and rest them on the floor. Gently drop your knees to the right side. Hold, and then roll your knees over to the left.

Palpate Your Piggies

Your feet deserve a break today since you've been stomping around in your cross-trainers all week. Take them off and pamper those tootsies. Sit down and cross your right leg over your left thigh. Massage your right foot with the thumbs of both hands. Press into all the fleshy parts of your foot, making circular, pressing motions with your thumbs. Then switch sides. For an especially invigorating rub, use one of the many brands of peppermint foot massage cream available on the market. It'll have you revived and hopping back onto your feet in no time!

Squeeze . . . Now Relax

Relaxing by creating tension and then letting it go is a stress-relief technique where you learn to progressively relax.

Lie on your back with your hands resting by your sides. Straighten your legs and relax your feet. Focus on each body part, starting from your feet and moving upward. Breathe deeply and tense each muscle as you travel mentally up your body. Squeeze your body part, and then exhale and let it go completely. As you move your way up, your lower body will start to feel heavy. Feel the floor support you completely. By the end, you should feel as if you're floating on a cloud.

Bathtub Stretch

Nothing soothes a tired body more than a warm bath. You can double up your bubbletime by sneaking in a hamstring stretch since the back of your legs are one of the most common areas of the body to get tight. Lie back against the tub with your right leg extended on the bottom, your left knee bent, foot flat. Lean your head back and rest it comfortably on the tubside. Slowly extend your left leg straight up and gently hold onto the back of your thigh with your hands. Rather than trying to pull your leg too close to your chest, aim to straighten the knee completely and push the heel up to the ceiling. You will probably have to move your leg farther out to straighten the leg. Hold the stretch and breathe deeply until you feel your hamstrings in the back of the thigh start to loosen. Then switch sides.

Do Something Fun for Someone Else

Play ball with the dog. Play Frisbee. Grab a shoelace and play with the cat. Grab some crayons and play with your niece, nephew, kid, or neighbor's kid. Go on a walk with grandma. Bringing a little joy into someone else's life is a great way to feel good.

Breathe Deeply

You can calm down an anxious mind and wind down an antsy body with deep breathing. Find a place where you can feel safe and warm and where you won't be disturbed. Sit in a comfortable position with your back lengthened. Cross your legs into a comfortable position, or extend them in front of you. Relax your hands by your sides and unclench your shoulders. Inhale slowly through your nose and fill up your lungs with air as if you were blowing up a big balloon. Breathe in through the back of your nostrils and make the process of drawing in air as effortless as possible. Fill up your lungs from the abdomen on up. Breathe in long and deep to the count of four. Hold the air in for a second or two, and then exhale through your nose. Empty the air first through the bottom of your lungs, then the middle, and finally the top. Hold the lungs empty for one or two seconds so that you are in no hurry to force your breathing. Allow your body, your breath, your mind, and your muscles to relax.

Uncrick That Crick in Your Neck

If you frequently get tense, tight, crampy spots in your neck muscles, try this stretch: Sit tall in a chair and clasp your hands behind your back. Lift your rib cage and raise your arms up slightly behind you. Roll your shoulders back and squeeze your shoulder blades together. Gently lower your chin in front and roll it from shoulder to shoulder, ear to ear. Stop at any tight spots and breathe deeply, holding the stretch until you feel the neck tension release. Finally, unclasp your hands and hug yourself to open up the shoulder blades and stretch out your upper back.

Shake Your Groove Thang

The body was meant to move, and music is its muse. Go into a room and lock the door. Close the drapes. Put on some soothing, slow music that you love. Close your eyes, feel the sound, and dance. This is no aerobic workout. This is a slow appreciation of your body and being.

Revive Flagging Energy

In the Eastern traditions of yoga, tai chi, and the martial arts, energy, also known as *chi,* is said to follow along channels in our body. It is believed that the energy levels can weaken or become too strong, which in turn can affect how relaxed we feel as well as how healthy and energetic we are.

Tai chi, one of the meditative martial arts, uses a series of slow movements to harmonize the energy flow. Try this basic tai chi position:

1. **Stand with your feet shoulder-width apart. Point your toes forward; hang your hands by your sides.**

2. **Stand tall and imagine that a cord is suspending your head. Feel your body lengthen and sink simultaneously.**

3. **Exhale and imagine a cup of warm water is being poured over your head. As it flows down your body — down the neck, shoulders, and chest — feel it melt your tight muscles. As it continues to trickle down your body, feel the warmth cover all your muscles until it finally spreads to your feet. Feel your feet push into the floor.**

4. **Inhale and allow the floor to push your body up, feeling the pressure push against the bottom of your feet.**

   Up until now your hands have been hanging by your sides. As you feel the warmth rise up again, allow your hands to float, palms down, and rise up in front of your thighs, then hips, then ribs, and then chest. At the end of this inhale, your elbows should be bent, arms held in front of your body, and hands at shoulder level.

5. **Exhale again and allow the elbows to sink as the back of your hands move inward closer to your body, then slowly fall like leaves down by your sides again.**

6. **Feel the head suspend; then as the warm water pours over you, allow your hips and body to sink again.**

7. **Repeat until you feel completely relaxed.**

Catch Some ZZZZZs

Turn off the tube, and give your mind and body what they really want: REM-rich nourishment. Go rest. Exercising is only a part of your overall road to physical improvement. As you sleep, your body recovers and becomes stronger. If you're having trouble sleeping, that could be a sign that you're doing more than cross-training, you could be overtraining. Rest and dwell in it.

Chapter 27

Ten Ways to Stick to It

*I*t's Friday and you've been working out every other day for the past couple of months. The last thing you want to do is lace up your cross-trainers, step foot on a treadmill, or look at a weight. In fact, squatting on the couch is as much butt work as you feel like doing. So how do you keep your body in motion when the thought of exercise makes you want to hang up your gym bag indefinitely?

You've got to fight the mental battle. Your greatest ally — and your greatest foe — is your mind. Let's face it, you're physically capable of exercising, but your mental motor has gone dead. Once the newness, glamour, and excitement of your cross-training plan has worn off, *continuing* to exercise and exercising when you just don't feel like it is going to be difficult. This is when you have to muster up the most energy, because you've reached drop-out crunch time.

Studies show that most people get busy or bored and quit within the first six months of a new program. That might be after four weeks for some, or after a valiant 5½ months for others. If you're feeling the lure of the sofa, then your time is now and you've got to win the war. The key to getting motivated is figuring out your fitness trigger.

Be aware that what motivates you will constantly change. In our exercise lives we've gone through times when hopping on a cardio machine, or running around the park, was a no-brainer (we simply would not, could not, bring ourselves to do it). During other periods, the ability to pedal while watching the CNN coverage of the political debates was actually something we looked forward to. Sometimes fitness classes sound like fun, and sometimes they sound like death. When you get a case of *specific activity*-phobia, just do something else. It's as simple as that.

Getting yourself out of bed, off the sofa, and out of the house is absolutely, undeniably the hardest part about exercising. Engage yourself in a mental debate when you're feeling unmotivated; think of all the reasons why you should. Remind yourself of your goal. Say it out loud. Then, before you can analyze yourself further, do something. Every little bit will help your reach your goal. It's *easy* to give an all out effort for a short time and exercise every day for a couple of weeks. In fact, many people seem to prefer a short obsessive period of exercise, rather than the adopt-it-into-your-lifestyle approach. The problem is, your results won't be permanent unless you keep it up. It's all about consistency. Having a few days off or eating too much occasionally will not matter in the long term. It all balances out. If you eat an entire chocolate cake you won't gain 10 pounds overnight. If you ate a chocolate cake every day for a month, you would. If you exercise very intensely for a few days and then stop, ultimately you'll have little effect on your body. If you exercise a little bit every day, ultimately you'll notice dramatic effects on your body. Forcing yourself to exercise is difficult. When you *naturally* want to, it all becomes effortless. The key is keeping yourself motivated so that you naturally want to.

We've racked our brains for all the things that have helped get us through our fitness downtimes. Here are some ideas to help you keep on movin' if you've found that you've started slowin' down.

A New Outfit Never Hurts

It's strange but true. Buying a new pair of cross-trainers, a new fitness bra, running pants, or thong leotard (if they're still your thing) can suddenly make you yearn for the gym. We don't know why, but the prospect of looking at ourselves, or having others look at ourselves, looking good in a new get-up is a good motivator. (Check out Appendix B for great fitness gear Web sites. It works like this: You can surf the sites while you're in couch-potato mode. When your order arrives, you emerge a motivated, new you!) If you're not the fashionable type, the principle still applies when it comes to fitness equipment. Accessorize: Purchase a new sports watch, pedometer, or a snazzy new helmet! You'll be raring to try them out!

Hook Up with Someone

For those of you who are tired of going to the park or gym alone, get yourself a training partner. A partner doubles your fun! More importantly, accountability makes it much harder to quit: You're responsible for your partner and he or she is responsible for you. Even if you don't feel like working out at the last minute, you're obligated to meet your partner because she is waiting for you. If you can't find a willing friend, put a notice up at your gym.

The Training-Partner Method isn't foolproof. Martica once met a friend at the park to go running. It was cold, and the six-mile run just didn't have the same appeal it usually did. Neither of them were in the mood, so they went for a pizza instead!

No Excuses on Lo-mo Days

You know what? Sometimes you have to get tough with yourself; crack the whip, just get out there, and do it. Exercise needs to become a habit, a normal part of your everyday life. If exercise is to create a lasting effect on your body, it must be continued, to some extent, forever. If you've ever had an evening where you're too tired to brush your teeth or remove your makeup, yet managed to drag yourself to the bathroom anyway, this is what you have to do during lo-mo (low motivation) days. Just do something, *anything,* for five minutes. Remember the exercise goals you made when you first started your program? Remember the smaller, subgoals you made in order to keep the expectation realistic? Well, downsize: Make your baby steps even smaller: Instead of a super-long session, halve it. Do just your biceps curls or simply jog in place for 10 or 15 minutes. Chances are you'll keep moving for longer. But even if you don't, something is better than nothing, and the next workout can now be five minutes shorter.

Record Your Progress

If you haven't been recording your exercise sessions, it's time to start. Keeping a journal will give you a sort of *gold star* mentality to help you keep on track. If you've been using our workout logs in Appendix C, chances are they've spurred you on up until now. But that doesn't mean that you don't need a fresh new page. Start again so that your plan feels new and exciting again — you might even want to re-evaluate your aims and progress with a whole new goal. But write it down: Seeing the proof of success helps motivation along.

 Martica has a romper-room approach that has worked well for her and her clients. All you need is a sheet or paper and a bright pink or yellow highlighter. Draw your own workout calendar, starting from the day you intend to start working out (like today) and extend it for about six weeks, filling in the appropriate days and dates. Then, each day you work out, fill in what you did: "ran 30 minutes" or "lifted weights and step class." Use a bright color to fill in the square. Pretty soon you'll have a whole calendar filled with happy squares! If you have too many white squares, you can immediately detect your dropout potential and get moving quick. Some days, the fact that you get to color a square in is enough to get you laced up and out the door.

Entertain Yourself

Whistling while you work can make the most gruesome of workouts a little more enjoyable, as can any sort of distraction. So use a Walkman when you run (on low volume, please, to protect your eardrums). Read a book or magazine when you're on a stationary bike or stair machine. And tune in because gym equipment with Internet, movie, and CD capabilities are coming to a gym near you.

Our favorite music pick-me-ups are

- Robbie Williams: *The Ego Has Landed.*

- Prince: *Greatest Hits.*

- Santana: *Supernatural.*

- Jamiroquai: *Traveling Without Moving.*

- Madonna: *Ray of Light.*

- Specially mixed fitness music used by professional fitness instructors. Try mixes from Power Productions, Muscle Mixes, Dynamix, and TelStar Fitness (see Appendix B for ordering information).

Give It Five Minutes

You may not feel like doing your usual hour-long workout on some days. Then don't. Cut the workout to 30 minutes, but really push yourself during that time. Or even give it five (see "No Excuses on Lo-mo Days"). If you can just convince yourself to do a little bit of something, you'll often find that you complete a whole workout anyway. Numerous studies show that high-intensity exercise programs have a higher drop-out rate. With limited time each day, it's impossible to stick to a compulsive exercise regimen. You end up neglecting other areas of your life. Fitter people have more of a problem doing short easy workouts because they feel like it's a waste of time if they don't do an hour and a half. It isn't.

Keep It Low, Go Slow

Stop looking for a miracle. One study showed that those who stuck with their exercise program saw it as a lifestyle change rather than a temporary pastime. The ones who stuck to it planned on working out about three times each week. The dropouts only expected to work out once a week. This alone would be enough to make most people quit, since the less exercise you do, the fewer benefits can be seen in a short time, discouraging you from continuing.

If you are a beginner or work out at an easy fitness level, realize that a low-intensity exercise takes longer to give results. But rather than get disappointed along the way, be patient. Results will come if you stick to it. If you're not satisfied with the results you're getting, re-evaluate your plan to see how you can make it more effective. Instead of berating yourself for finishing your workout early, or even taking a day off, focus on what you've accomplished instead. Recognize the stages you'll go through. Initially you will have hopes of your success, you will be enthusiastic and believe that you can do it. As you become more experienced, you'll start taking a more strategical perspective; over time you'll develop confidence and toughness that will let you push yourself more.

Get High

Exercise releases pleasure hormones. You'll feel good even on minimal amounts of any types of physical activity, from yoga and deep breathing to running and football, and any vigorous exercise can leave you feeling happy and exhilarated after even a short time. But to experience what is known as an *aerobic high,* where the brain is awash in feel-good endorphins, studies indicate that you must do *intense* exercise for an extended period of time. If you've reached this point, you could suddenly feel as if you're running on air and exerting no effort at all. If you're fit enough to do so, push yourself to reach this high.

Reassess Your Goal

If you're in a rut, you might need a new goal. Take a good look at what you've achieved and insert a new dose of cross-training into your schedule. (Check out Chapter 4 for a refresher on goal-setting.)

You can also splurge on a personal trainer once a month or once every six months to help revamp your routine. You can hire a trainer privately or at most health clubs for $25-$85 per session. Split the cost with a friend if you find it out of your range. You might just find that you learn little tips and tidbits about your workout that can motivate you to new levels of commitment — with better results.

Take a Break

If you're really burned out, take time off to vegetate and rejuvenate. Chances are you need this relaxation time. The amount of sleep you have had, your mood, diet, and any stress you're under can affect your energy levels. If you're not getting enough nutrients or enough calories, your body may not function efficiently and you'll feel tired and listless. Eat plenty of fruit, vegetables, and other carbohydrates to fuel your energy levels.

When you are ready to take exercise by storm once again, you'll be refreshed and ready to go. It's fine to miss a few days in your schedule every now and then. It won't harm your long-term goal as long as your overall participation is consistent.

Chapter 28

Ten Great Bench Stretches

- -

In This Chapter

▶ Using a bench to position yourself into comfortable stretches

▶ Lengthening the muscles in your upper and lower body

- -

*T*ake a long, deep breath, and get ready to relax because we've created a total-body stretching sequence that will help you chill out and loosen up. You can roll up your exercise mat, because instead of plopping you on the floor, we've hoisted you up onto a bench. Being on an elevated platform allows you to dangle your legs in different positions to maneuver into a variety of deep, satisfying stretches. You can do this head-to-toe routine on a bench at the gym or on your sofa or bed at home. Do the whole series as one fluid sequence on one side and then repeat on the other side. Or do each stretch, alternating both sides before moving on. Hold each position for 10-60 seconds.

If a muscle feels strained, or any part of your body feels uncomfortable, you may have pushed too far: Back up and decrease the range of motion of your stretch. Check our safety tips for ways to modify stressful positions.

Hip and Thigh Bench Stretch

You'll feel this stretch in the quadriceps and hip flexors of your back leg. You might also feel a stretch in the calf and Achilles tendon, or the hamstrings of the front leg (see Figure 28-1).

1. **Stand in front of a bench or chair, and place your right foot on the seat. Hands are on your hips.**

2. **Bend your right knee to 90 degrees. Extend the back leg behind you and bend the back knee slightly. Press your right hip forward.**

3. **Hold, and then switch legs.**

Safety Tip: If your rear calf feels strained, lift your back heel off the ground.

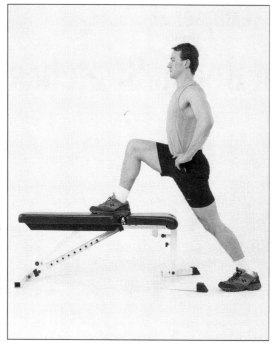

Figure 28-1:
In this stretch, you lengthen the front of your straight leg.

Hamstring and Quad Bench Stretch

Your thighs get a double whammy with this stretch (see Figure 28-2). Here, you feel the tension release both in the hamstrings in the back of your straight leg on the bench and in the quadriceps in the front of the lowered thigh.

1. **Stand facing the end of the bench, and place your right foot on top. Slide that foot forward down the length of the bench so your leg is completely outstretched and supported. Your hips are now centered over the middle of the bench, right leg on top, left leg to the left side.**

2. **Lower your body so that you are sitting on the bench with your leg extended. Your left leg should hang off the side.**

3. **Bend the left knee just underneath your left hip, and curl the toe under, keeping your foot behind your hips. Sit up straight and hold the position. Then switch sides.**

Safety Tip: If your back knee feels strained, move your leg forward so that the leg is bent in front of your body, foot flat on the floor.

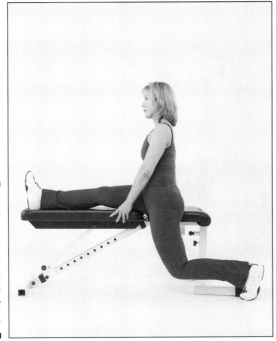

Figure 28-2:
Keep your spine straight and back lifted as you stretch the back of your front leg.

Hamstring Bench Stretch

You focus on the back of your straight leg in this stretch (see Figure 28-3). After you feel the hamstrings in the back thigh relax, straighten your knee and flex your front foot to increase the stretch to the lower leg.

1. **Sit straddling a bench with your right leg extended straight in front of you on the top of the bench.**

2. **Place your left leg on the left side with the knee bent and foot flat on the ground.**

3. **Lift your rib cage and lean slightly forward to press your chest towards your top thigh.**

   Don't worry about touching your head or chest to your knees because that may cause you to round and strain your lower back. Instead, hold your chest high and press your lower back toward the front thigh.

4. **Press your knee down to straighten leg. Then switch sides.**

Safety Tip: If your straight leg feels tight, soften your knee.

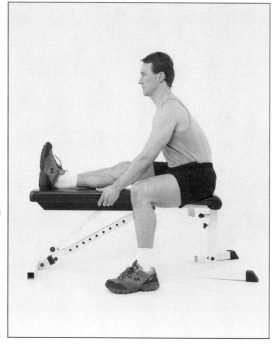

Figure 28-3:
Lean forward from your hip joint instead of bending at the waist.

Calf and Chest

We flip you to your other side in a position similar to the hamstring stretch in Figure 28-3. We evolve the movement to include a pectoral stretch for your chest and a deeper leg stretch to target your gastrocnemius in the calf (see Figure 28-4).

1. **Sit sideways on a bench, facing the end, with your left leg extended straight in front of you on the bench.**

2. **Place your right leg off the side with the knee bent and foot flat on the ground.**

3. **Clasp your hands behind your back, raise your arms, and open your shoulders to stretch your chest.**

4. **At the same time, lift your rib cage and lean slightly toward your straight leg as you move your right toe toward your body to stretch the calf. Hold, then relax your foot and arms and then switch sides.**

Safety Tip: If this stretch is too intense in the calf, relax your flexed foot.

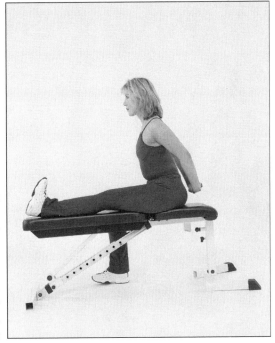

Figure 28-4:
Remember
to exhale
as you
stretch
to help
relax your
muscles.

Back, Neck, and Outer Thigh Bench Stretch

Shifting your body in slightly different directions during a stretch can help you target different areas of a muscle. This stretch will loosen up your hamstrings along with your back, neck, and outer thigh (see Figure 28-5).

1. **Sit sideways on a bench facing the end with your left leg extended straight on top. Place your right leg off the side, knee bent, foot flat on the ground.**

2. **Holding your torso high, rotate your upper body slightly to the left, placing both hands on the outside of your left thigh on the edge of the bench.**

3. **Lower your shoulders and turn the neck as far as you comfortably can. Hold, and then switch sides.**

Safety Tip: Don't force your body into an extreme twist.

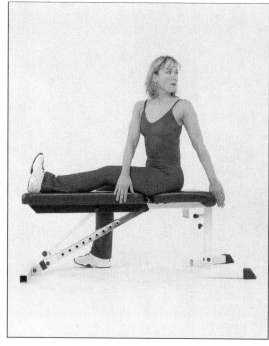

Figure 28-5:
Imagine a string pulling your head and rib cage higher and farther away from your hips.

Inner Thigh and Spine Bench Stretch

Your inner thigh muscles and lower back will thank you for this little number. Maintain perfect posture and allow your body to relax as you perform this stretch (see Figure 28-6).

1. **Sit sideways on a bench with your right leg extended straight on the bench. Place your left leg off the side, knee bent, foot flat on the ground. Open your left knee and foot so that your inner thighs are wide apart.**

2. **Rotate your upper body toward the left, placing your hands on the outside of the left thigh.**

3. **Use your right hand for leverage against the outer left knee to increase the spinal twist. Avoid sinking into your lower back; sit tall.**

4. **Look over your left shoulder and keep your chin level with the floor. Hold, and then switch sides.**

Safety Tip: If you feel strain in your inner knee of the straight leg, move your legs closer together. If your back feels strained, decrease the rotation outward.

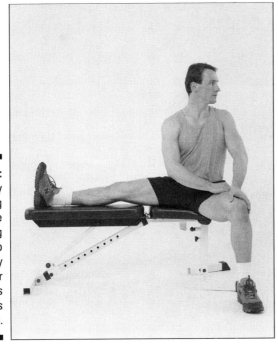

Figure 28-6:
Sit tall by lengthening your spine and holding your rib cage away from your pelvis during this stretch.

Side Torso Bench Stretch

Ready to loosen up your upper body? We add a back, abs, and chest stretch to this lower body move (see Figure 28-7).

1. **Sit sideways on a bench with your right leg extended straight on top of the bench. Place your left leg off the side, knee bent, foot flat on the ground. Turn the left knee outward to separate the thighs.**

2. **Face your left knee. With your left hand on your left leg, raise your right arm overhead and lift your rib cage to stretch out your torso.**

3. **Lean slightly to the left. Relax your neck, and open your chest towards the ceiling. Drop your right shoulder slightly down in front. Switch sides.**

Safety Tip: Rather than bend your back too far sideways, lift up to elongate the spine.

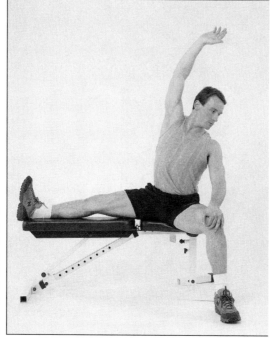

Figure 28-7:
Tony is working his upper and lower body with this stretch.

Inner Thigh and Gluteals Stretch

You'll feel this stretch in the back, at the back of the right hip and inner thigh, and in your buttocks. Allow your upper body to sink toward the lower body in this move (see Figure 28-8).

1. **Sitting sideways on a bench facing the end, hang your right leg off the side and bend your left knee on top of the bench so the left thigh rotates out.**

2. **Lengthen your spine, then lean forward and lower your head and shoulders. Hold onto the front of the bench to support the weight of your upper body.**

3. **If you feel pressure in your lower back, try not to bend over, instead raise your ribs higher.**

Safety Tip: If your right knee feels strained, move the right foot down the bench closer to your calf to open the knee to a wider angle.

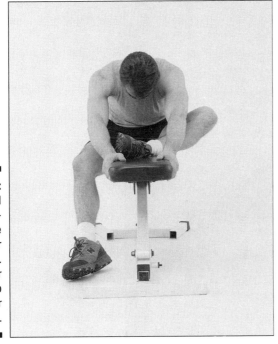

Figure 28-8:
Avoid
pulling your-
self to force
a deeper
stretch.
Allow your
muscles to
relax at their
own pace.

Hip Bench Stretch

Once you're feeling flexible, you can shift into this lunge to target the front of your back thigh. The bench will help support the weight of your upper body.

1. **Sitting sideways straddling a bench facing the end, place your right leg on the right side, knee bent, foot flat. Slide your left leg underneath and behind you so that it extends — knee facing down — in back.**

2. **Make sure your right knee is bent in a lunge position at a 90-degree angle in front of your body. Left toe and knee should both point forward.**

3. **Place your left hand on the bench inside your right knee for support.**

4. **Hold your ribs high and press your left hip down. Press your chest forward. If your back feels strained from being arched, lean your straight spine slightly forward.**

Safety Tip: If this stretch feels too extreme in the hip, raise your torso up slightly or perform the move in a standing lunge position (see Figure 28-9).

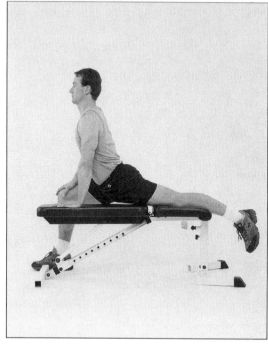

Figure 28-9:
You can modify this stretch if it pushes you too far by raising your hips higher.

Neck, Upper Back, and Gluteals Bench Stretch

If you store tension in your shoulders and upper back, you'll enjoy this final stretch that also targets your inner thighs and buttocks. Sit tall and exhale to help release the tight muscles (see Figure 28-10).

1. **Cross both your legs so that you sit Indian-style on top of the bench.**

2. **Gently place your hands against the back of your head and sit up straight, slightly pulling your chin toward your chest. Lean slightly forward to shift your body weight in front of your hips, but avoid bending at your waist.**

3. **To target more of the upper back, bring your elbows forward and round your upper back slightly to separate the shoulder blades.**

4. **To stretch more of the neck, sit tall and release your hands. Drop your ear to your right shoulder and then repeat on the other side.**

Safety Tip: Avoid putting too much pressure on your head with your hands. Try not to allow your lower back to sink. Instead, think of rising up and expanding your upper back.

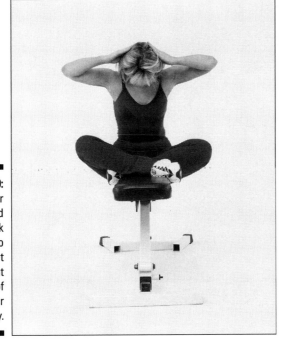

Figure 28-10:
Shift your arm and back position to target different areas of your upper body.

Part VII
Appendixes

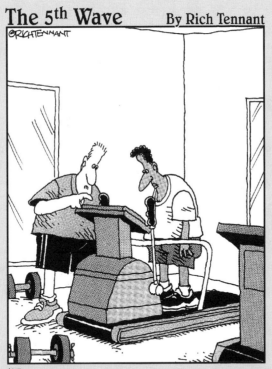

The 5th Wave   By Rich Tennant

"This readout shows your heart rate, blood pressure, bone density, skin hydration, plaque buildup, liver function, and expected lifetime!"

In this part . . .

We include resources to find more information about videos, fitness organizations, fitness equipment, and so on. Also, the workout log can help you track your progress, while the glossary will give you terms to throw around at the gym to make you feel less a fitness dummy.

Appendix A

Glossary

abduction: Moving a limb away from your body, such as in a standing side leg lift.

adduction: Moving a limb towards your body, such as when closing your arm in a fly.

atrophy: A loss of muscle tissue.

ballistic stretching: Pulsing or bouncing during a stretch; this technique increases the risk of injury from overstretching.

biceps: An abbreviated term for the biceps brachii muscle.

biceps brachii: The muscle in the front of the upper arm that helps bend your elbow.

brachialis: The muscle in the front of the upper arm that helps to flex the elbow when your forearm is rotated outward.

brachioradialis: The muscle in the arm that helps bend your elbow when the forearm is at the midpoint between being rotated inward and outward.

carbohydrates: The food source that is converted to fat or glycogen; sources of fuel that the body uses to produce energy.

concentric phase: When a muscle contracts to move the bones it is attached to, it exerts force and shortens. This is usually the initial and most forceful phase of a lift (the bending part of a biceps curl, for example).

cooldown: The post-exercise phase of a workout, where you gradually decrease the intensity of a vigorous workout to a low intensity.

cross-trainers: The style of fitness training shoe that is designed to be worn during a variety of general activities as opposed to a specialist shoe that is created for the movement patterns of a particular sport.

cross-training: The practice of incorporating a variety of modes of exercise into an overall training program, or of doing several types of activity during one exercise session.

deltoids: Muscles around the shoulder joint that raise up the arms.

eccentric phase: Following the concentric phase, the muscle remains slightly contracted as it lengthens to move the bones (and weight) back to the original position. This return, or eccentric, phase, also known as a negative contraction, is aided by gravitational pull. Make sure to slow down during this portion of your lift.

endurance training: Doing cardiovascular exercise such as running, cycling, or rowing to improve oxygen consumption and the ability to exercise for long periods of time.

erector spinae: The long muscle running along the spine that branches, attaching to ribs and vertebrae. It bends the spine sideways or moves from a bent to erect position. (Other smaller muscles also assist in bending and straightening the spine.)

extension: Opening a joint so that its angle increases, such as when arching your back or straightening your knee.

Fartlek training: Coined from a Swedish word that means "speed play," a method of training for endurance activities during which a continuous training period is broken up with high-intensity intervals and lower-intensity relief periods.

fast twitch: One of two distinct types of muscle fibers that are associated with high-energy, fast contractions such as those needed for power lifting and sprinting.

flexion: When a joint is bent so that its angle decreases. When doing an ab curl or bending your knee, you're contracting a muscle to flex the joint.

gastrocnemius: The bulging muscle on the calves that points your toes and allows you to rise up on your toes.

glutes, gluteals: A short term for the muscle group in the buttocks that includes the gluteus maximus, gluteus medius, and gluteus minimus.

gluteus maximus: The largest of the muscles in your buttocks. It extends your leg behind you and rotates your thigh outward. This muscle gives the buttocks its shape.

gluteus medius: Another buttocks muscle that moves the leg away from the body, as well as rotates the thigh inward.

gluteus minimus: This muscle lies underneath the gluteus medius and mainly rotates the thigh inward.

hamstrings: The group of three muscles in the back thigh that bend the knee joint: the semimembranosus, the semitendinosus, and the biceps femoris, which is the most powerful of the hamstring muscles.

high-intensity exercise: Doing cardiovascular or strength exercise at a level that pushes yourself beyond a moderate level of exertion, such as sprinting instead of walking.

hip flexors: A common term for the muscles in the front of the hip that raise the thigh, the iliopsoas.

hyperextension: Continuing to open a joint past its neutral position, such as when locking a joint.

hyperflexion: Closing a joint angle to the extreme, such as when doing a deep knee bend.

inner thigh group: Five muscles that help flex the hip, bring the thigh across the body, and rotate the thigh inward. These include the pectineus, adductor brevis, adductor longus, adductor magnus, and gracilis.

interval training: A method of alternating very high-intensity bouts of activity with rest periods. The intervals can range from a few seconds to a few minutes in duration.

lactate threshold: The level of exertion during cardiovascular exercise where the amount of the waste product of metabolism, lactic acid, builds up faster than it is eliminated. Becoming fitter raises this threshold, allowing you to work harder.

latissimus dorsi: This broad muscle covers most of the middle and lower back; it brings arms close to the body. It also rotates the upper arm inward.

levator scapulae: This muscle connects the shoulder blades and neck. It elevates, rotates, and draws the shoulder blades in.

ligament: Connective tissue that links bones to each other.

lo-mo days: Slang term for low motivation days, those times when you simply do not feel inspired to exercise.

max VO2: Aerobic capacity, or the highest amount of oxygen that the body can use during high-intensity exercise. It increases the fitter you become.

muscle fiber: A single muscle cell. Muscle fibers in the eye can be just a few millimeters long, while large skeletal muscle fibers in the leg can be 100mm long.

obliques: Abdominal muscles that twist your torso. They span diagonally from the ribs to the hips. The two layers are the internal and external obliques.

periodization: A way of organizing your long-term workout plan into cycles so that you hone in on improving different areas of fitness during each period.

PNF stretching: Proprioceptive Neuromuscular Facilitation stretching; a technique of contracting a muscle with resistance prior to stretching it.

pyramid sets: Using gradually heavier or lighter loads on a muscle group during one set of reps or between sets.

quadratus lumborum: The muscle running along the lower spine. When fibers from both sides contract, the spine is stabilized; when one side contracts, the spine bends.

quadriceps femoris: The group of four muscles along the front of the thigh that straighten the knee.

quads: Short term for the quadriceps muscle group in the front thigh.

range of motion: The expanse of movement through which a joint can move. The standard range of motion (ROM) for the knee joint is from a fully bent to a fully straight 180-degree angle. Stretching a muscle increases the ROM of a joint.

rectus abdominis: The muscle that runs down the center of your torso, from the lower ribs to the pelvic bones. When flexed, it bends your trunk at the waist and ripples to create the "six-pack" look.

rectus femoris: Located in the center of the upper half of the thigh. It flexes the hip and extends the knee.

Repetition Maximum (RM): The most weight one muscle group can lift in one repetition. Measuring this can help you monitor strength changes over time.

resistance: A force that inhibits the motion of a muscle resulting in a slowing effect during a movement. Weights, rubber bands, body weight, and even the water when swimming, all provide resistance for the muscles to work against.

resting heart rate: The number of heartbeats per minute when the body is at rest. Best taken upon first waking in the morning. Endurance athletes can have resting heart rates of 35-50; the average person may range from 60-80. A lower resting heart rate often reflects a greater cardiovascular efficiency.

rhomboids: This muscle lies between the shoulder blades. When contracted, it elevates and brings them together.

RPE (Rate of Perceived Exertion): A scale first devised by Swedish Professor Gunnar Borg to rate the level of effort you feel during exercise. The current scale being used is a 10-point scale, with 0 meaning that very little or no effort is felt and 10 indicating that the effort is of an extremely high intensity.

serratus anterior: This muscle lies on the outer ribs, underneath the armpits. It opens and depresses the shoulder blades.

set: A group of single repetitions of an exercise; although most routines include up to four sets, research shows that 80 percent of strength is gained from doing one set only.

slow twitch: One of two types of muscle fibers that prefer aerobic metabolism and are recruited for slower, low-intensity, endurance activities, such as walking or moderate-paced cycling.

soleus: Muscle that lies beneath the gastrocnemius and assists in pointing the toe.

split routine: Alternating upper and lower body exercises on different days, rather than doing a routine that targets the whole body each workout.

sprain: When a ligament is torn.

static stretching: Holding a stretch very still, without bouncing.

strain: When a muscle or tendon is injured but not torn.

strength training: Using resistance to increase muscle strength.

stretch reflex: A mechanism where muscle fibers will shorten in order to protect against being overstretched. Further stretching past this tightening may cause injury to the muscles. If a stretch hurts, decrease the range of motion to prevent this response.

super sets: Either performing two different exercises consecutively for the same muscle group (for example, a lat pulldown and then a bentover row) or doing two exercises for the same body part but working opposing muscles (a biceps curl followed by a triceps dip).

Target Heart Rate: The number of heartbeats per minute that will elicit desired training effects such as improved aerobic and anaerobic capacity.

tendon: The fibrous tissue that connects the muscle to a bone.

tensor fasciae latae: Muscle on the outer thigh that flexes and moves the thigh away from the body.

torque: Rotation or twisting of a joint.

transversus abdominis: Deepest abdominal muscle located in the lower torso that compresses the contents of the abdominal wall.

trapezius: This muscle covers most of the upper back. It returns your arms toward your body when they are extended and also brings your shoulder blades together.

triceps: The short term for the triceps brachii muscle in the upper arm.

triceps brachii: The muscle in the back of the upper arm that straightens the elbow.

vastus intermedius: Muscle located in the upper thigh. It helps, along with the rectus femoris, to stabilize the leg when standing.

vastus lateralis: A muscle on the outer front thigh.

vastus medialis: The most active muscle in the quad group that lies on the lower part of the inner front thigh. It also helps prevent dislocation of the kneecap. All three vasti muscles are most active during the final degrees of straightening the knee.

warm up: The process of slowly raising your heart rate and body temperature at the beginning of an exercise session in preparation to stretch or work up to a higher intensity.

Appendix B

Resources

● ●

*T*hroughout this book we mention special equipment, such as stability balls, for use in your training. This appendix provides you with resources to find stability balls and other useful fitness equipment. We also point you to home gym equipment, cross-training shoes, fitness clothing, fitness and nutrition organizations on the Web, and amateur sports associations.

Fitness Tools and Equipment

For information on Martica's books and videos, look up www.Amazon.co.uk, www.Amazon.com, www.BarnesandNoble.com, or send a self-addressed stamped envelope to Martica's Fitness Products, P.O. Box 2034, New York City, NY 10021.

Collage Video, 5390 Main St. N.E., Minneapolis, MN 55421, phone 1-800-433-6769; web site www.collagevideo.com. Collage Video offers virtually tons of aerobics videos and other fitness classes on videotapes.

Fitness Wholesale, 895-A Hampshire Rd., Stow, OH 44224; phone 1-800-537-5512 or 330-929-7227; web site www.fitnesswholesale.com. Fitness Wholesale offers products you're likely to see in your local gym, including stability balls, rubber bands, and steps.

Flexaball, P.O. Box 33536, Indialantic, FL 32903; phone 1-800-413-9942; fax 321-674-9914; web site www.megafitness.com. This giant web site offers just about any piece of equipment you've "seen on TV" — from gadgets to really good stuff.

Polar Electro, Inc., 370 Crossways Park Dr., Woodbury, NY 11797-2050; phone 1-800-227-1314; fax 516-364-5454; web site www.polarusa.com. Polar Electro makes heart rate monitors — some of the best in the business!

SPRI Products, Inc., 1584 Barclay Blvd., Buffalo Grove, IL 60089; phone 1-800-222-7774; web site www.spriproducts.com. You can get Resist-A-Ball and a variety of other fitness equipment from this one site.

The Step Company, 400 Interstate N. Parkway, Suite 1500, Atlanta, GA 30339; phone 1-800-729-7837.

Resist-A-Ball, 6435 Castleway W. Dr., Suite 130, Indianapolis, IN 46250; phone 1-800-843-3671. Resist-A-Ball provides stability balls, which are great for working your abs.

Rollerblade Inc., 5101 Shady Oak Rd., Minnetonka, MN 55343; phone 1-800-328-0171; web site www.rollerblade.com. Check out this web site for the popular in-line skating gear from Rollerblade.

JustBalls, web site www.justballs.com. This web site offers — you guessed it — just balls! You can find basketballs, footballs, softballs, and so on.

Home Gym Equipment

Concept II, R.R. 1, Box 1100, Morrisville, VT 05661; phone 1-800-245-5676; web site www.ConceptII.com.

Landice Inc., 111 Canfield Ave., Randolph, NJ 07869-1114; phone 1-800-LANDICE; web site www.landice.com.

Life Fitness, 10601 Belmont Ave., Franklin Park, IL 60131-1545, phone 1-800-735-3867; web site www.lifefitness.com.

Gym Source, 40 East 52nd St., New York City, NY 10022; phone 1-800-gym-source or 212-688-4222; web site www.gymsource.com.

Keiser Corporation, 2470 South Cherry Ave., Fresno, CA 93706; phone 1-800-888-7009; web site www.keiser.com.

Precor, Inc., 20001 North Creek Pkwy, P.O. Box 3004, Bothell, WA 98041; phone 1-800-786-8404; web site www.precor.com.

Schwinn Cycling & Fitness Inc., 1690 38th St., Boulder, CO 80301; phone 1-800-SCHWINN; web site www.schwinn.com.

StairMaster, 12421 Willows Rd. NE, Suite 100, Kirkland, WA 98034; phone 1-800-635-2936; web site www.stairmaster.com.

StarTrac by Unisen, Inc., 14410 Myford Rd., Irvine, CA 92606; phone 1-800-228-6635 or 714-669-1660; web site www.startrac.com.

Tunturi, Sta-Fit Gym Equipment, 1004 S.W. 10th St., Aledo, IL 61231-2353; phone 309-582-5334; web site www.tunturi.com.

Versiclimber, Heart Rate Inc., 3188 Airway Ave. #E, Costa Mesa, CA 92626-6601; phone 1-800-237-2271.

York Barbell, P.O. Box 1707, York, PA 17405; phone 1-800-358-YORK; web site www.yorkbarbell.com.

Cross-trainers and Other Sports Shoes

Adidas, P.O. Box 4015, Beaverton, OR 97076-4015; phone 503-972-2300; web site www.adidas.com.

Asics, 10540 Talbert Ave., Fountain Valley, CA 92708; phone 1-800-678-9435; web site www.asicstiger.com.

AVIA, 9605 S.W. Nimbus Ave., Beaverton, OR 97008; phone 1-800-345-2842; web site www.aviashoes.com.

NIKE, One Bowerman Dr., Beaverton, OR 97005; phone 1-800-806-6453; web site www.nike.com.

Reebok, 100 Technology Center Dr., Stoughton, MA 02072; phone 617-341-5000; web site www.reebok.com.

Rockport, 220 Donald Lynch Blvd., Marlborough, MA 01752; phone 1-800-762-5767; web site www.rockport.com.

Ryka, 555 South Henderson Rd., King of Prussia, PA 19406-3514; phone 1-800-255-RYKA; web site www.ryka.com.

New Balance Athletic Shoe, 61 N. Beacon St., Boston, MA 02134; phone 1-800-NBF-STOR; web site www.newbalance.com.

Saucony, P.O. Box 6046, Peabody, MA, 01960; phone 1-800-365-7282; web site www.saucony.com.

Fitness and Nutrition Organizations

Aerobics & Fitness Association of America (AFAA), 15250 Ventura Blvd., Suite 310, Sherman Oaks, CA 91403; phone 818-905-0040.

American College of Sports Medicine (ACSM), P.O. Box 1440, Indianapolis, IN 46206-1440; phone 317-637-9200; web site www.acsm.org.

American Council on Exercise, P.O. Box 910449, San Diego, CA 92191-0049; phone 1-800-825-3636 or 858-535-8227; web site www.acefitness.org.

American Dietetic Association, 216 West Jackson Blvd., #800, Chicago, IL 60606-6995; phone 1-800-877-1600.

Cooper Institute for Aerobics Research, 12330 Preston Rd, Dallas, TX 75230; phone 1-800-635-7050; web site www.cooperinst.org.

IDEA — The Association for Fitness Professionals, Suite 204, 6190 Cornerstone Ct. East, San Diego, California 92121-3773; phone 858-535-8979; web site www.ideafit.com.

National Academy of Sports Medicine, 699 Hampshire Rd., Suite 105, Westlake Village, CA 91361; phone 805-449-1330.

National Strength and Conditioning Association, P.O. Box 38909, Colorado Springs, CO 80937-8909.

Women's Sports Foundation, 342 Madison Ave., Suite 728, New York City, NY 10173; phone 212-972-9170.

Associations for Sporting Activities

Ironman World Triathlon Corporation, 1570 U.S. Highway 19 North, Tarpon Springs, FL 34689; phone 813-943-4767; web site www.ironmanlive.com.

Road Runners Clubs of America, 629 S. Washington St., Alexandria, VA 22314; phone 703-836-0558; web site www.rrca.org.

Triathlon Federation USA, P.O. Box 15820, Colorado Springs, CO 80935-5820; phone 719-597-9090.

United States Cycling Federation, 1750 East Boulder St., Colorado Springs, CO 80909; phone 719-578-4581; web site www.adventuresports.com/asap/uscf/uscf.htm.

United States Masters Swimming, 2 Peter Ave., Rutland, MA 01543; phone 508-886-6631; web site www.usms.org.

United States Swimming, 1750 East Boulder St., Colorado Springs, CO 80909; 719-578-4578; web site www.usswim.org.

USA Track and Field, P.O. Box 120, Indianapolis, IN 46206; phone 317-261-0500.

Appendix C

Workout Logs

- -

We provide three workout logs in this appendix that you can use to chart your progress on a daily, weekly, monthly, and even yearly schedule.

Weekly Log

Record your weekly exercise activity, following these directions:

- ✔ **Cardio:** Record the activities, the duration per session, and your level of intensity
- ✔ **Strength:** Record the name/number of the exercises that you will do, the number of sets and reps, and the amount of weight used
- ✔ **Flexibility:** Record the number of sessions per week and the duration per session
- ✔ **Power:** Record the name/number of the exercises that you do, the number of sets and reps and/or time duration, and the number of sessions per week
- ✔ **Skills:** Record the name/number of the drills that you do, the number of sets and reps and/or time duration, and the number of sessions per week

Table C-1

Weekly Log for Week Beginning _____

	Monday	Tuesday	Wednesday	Thursday	Friday	Saturday	Sunday	Weekly Comments
CARDIO STAMINA								
Activity: _____ Duration Intensity								
Activity: _____ Duration Intensity								
Activity: _____ Duration Intensity								
Activity: _____ Duration Intensity								
Activity: _____ Duration Intensity								
MUSCLE STRENGTH								
Exercise: _____ Weight Sets/reps								

	Monday	Tuesday	Wednesday	Thursday	Friday	Saturday	Sunday	Weekly Comments
Exercise: _____ Weight _____ Sets/reps								
Exercise: _____ Weight _____ Sets/reps								
Exercise: _____ Weight _____ Sets/reps								
Exercise: _____ Weight _____ Sets/reps								
Exercise: _____ Weight _____ Sets/reps								
Exercise: _____ Weight _____ Sets/reps								
Exercise: _____ Weight _____ Sets/reps								
Exercise: _____ Weight _____ Sets/reps								

(continued)

Table C-1 (continued)

	Monday	Tuesday	Wednesday	Thursday	Friday	Saturday	Sunday	Weekly Comments
Exercise: _____ Weight Sets/reps **FLEXIBILITY**								
Activity/Duration **POWER**								
Exercise: _____ Time Sets/reps								
Exercise: _____ Time Sets/reps								
Exercise: _____ Time Sets/reps								
Exercise: _____ Time Sets/reps								

	Monday	Tuesday	Wednesday	Thursday	Friday	Saturday	Sunday	Weekly Comments
Exercise: _____ Time _____ Sets/reps								
Exercise: _____ Time _____ Sets/reps								
SKILLS								
Activity: _____ Time _____ Sets/reps								
Activity: _____ Time _____ Sets/reps								
Activity: _____ Time _____ Sets/reps								
Activity: _____ Time _____ Sets/reps								
Activity: _____ Time _____ Sets/reps								
Activity: _____ Time _____ Sets/reps								

Tri-Monthly Plan

This schedule allows you to have an overview of your 120-week plan. You can plan and see your progression from month to month. Here is what you should include in the chart.

- ✔ **Cardio:** Record the activities you will do, the duration, and the number of sessions per week
- ✔ **Muscle Strength:** Record the name/number of the exercises that you will do, the number of sets and reps, and amount of weight used
- ✔ **Flexibility:** Record the number of sessions per week
- ✔ **Power:** Record the name/number of the exercises that you do, the number of sets and reps and/or time duration, and the number of sessions per week
- ✔ **Skills:** Record the name/number of the drills that you do, the number of sets and reps and/or time duration, and the number of sessions per week

Table C-2	Tri-monthly Log for Month Beginning _____		
	Month 1	**Month 2**	**Month 3**
Week 1			
CARDIO STAMINA			
Activity: _____ Duration Intensity			
Activity: _____ Duration Intensity			
Activity: _____ Duration Intensity			
MUSCLE STRENGTH			

	Month 1	Month 2	Month 3
Exercise: _____ Weight Sets/reps			
Exercise: _____ Weight Sets/reps			
Exercise: _____ Weight Sets/reps			
Exercise: _____ Weight Sets/reps			
Exercise: _____ Weight Sets/reps			
Exercise: _____ Weight Sets/reps			
Exercise: _____ Weight Sets/reps			
Exercise: _____ Weight Sets/reps			
Exercise: _____ Weight Sets/reps			
Exercise: _____ Weight Sets/reps			
Exercise: _____ Weight Sets/reps			
FLEXIBILITY			

(continued)

Table C-2 *(continued)*

	Month 1	Month 2	Month 3
POWER			
Exercise: _____ Time Sets/reps			
Exercise: _____ Time Sets/reps			
Exercise: _____ Time Sets/reps			
Exercise: _____ Time Sets/reps			
Exercise: _____ Time Sets/reps			
Skills			
Activity: _____ Time Sets/reps			
Activity: _____ Time Sets/reps			
Activity: _____ Time Sets/reps			
Activity: _____ Time Sets/reps			
Activity: _____ Time Sets/reps			

	Month 1	Month 2	Month 3
Week 2			
CARDIO STAMINA			
Activity: _____ Duration Intensity			
Activity: _____ Duration Intensity			
Activity: _____ Duration Intensity			
MUSCLE STRENGTH			
Exercise: _____ Weight Sets/reps			
Exercise: _____ Weight Sets/reps			
Exercise: _____ Weight Sets/reps			
Exercise: _____ Weight Sets/reps			
Exercise: _____ Weight Sets/reps			
Exercise: _____ Weight Sets/reps			

(continued)

Table C-2 *(continued)*

	Month 1	Month 2	Month 3
Exercise: _____ Weight Sets/reps			
Exercise: _____ Weight Sets/reps			
Exercise: _____ Weight Sets/reps			
Exercise: _____ Weight Sets/reps			
Exercise: _____ Weight Sets/reps			
FLEXIBILITY			
POWER			
Exercise: _____ Time Sets/reps			
Exercise: _____ Time Sets/reps			
Exercise: _____ Time Sets/reps			
Exercise: _____ Time Sets/reps			
Exercise: _____ Time Sets/reps			

	Month 1	Month 2	Month 3
SKILLS Checklist ✓ Easy ✓ Medium ✓ Difficult			
Activity: _____ Time Sets/reps			
Activity: _____ Time Sets/reps			
Activity: _____ Time Sets/reps			
Activity: _____ Time Sets/reps			
Activity: _____ Time Sets/reps			
Week 3			
CARDIO STAMINA			
Activity: _____ Duration Intensity			
Activity: _____ Duration Intensity			
Activity: _____ Duration Intensity			
MUSCLE STRENGTH			

(continued)

Table C-2 (continued)

	Month 1	Month 2	Month 3
Exercise: _____ Weight Sets/reps			
Exercise: _____ Weight Sets/reps			
Exercise: _____ Weight Sets/reps			
Exercise: _____ Weight Sets/reps			
Exercise: _____ Weight Sets/reps			
Exercise: _____ Weight Sets/reps			
Exercise: _____ Weight Sets/reps			
Exercise: _____ Weight Sets/reps			
Exercise: _____ Weight Sets/reps			
Exercise: _____ Weight Sets/reps			
Exercise: _____ Weight Sets/reps			
FLEXIBILITY			

	Month 1	Month 2	Month 3
POWER			
Exercise: _____ Time Sets/reps			
Exercise: _____ Time Sets/reps			
Exercise: _____ Time Sets/reps			
Exercise: _____ Time Sets/reps			
Exercise: _____ Time Sets/reps			
SKILLS			
Activity: _____ Time Sets/reps			
Activity: _____ Time Sets/reps			
Activity: _____ Time Sets/reps			
Activity: _____ Time Sets/reps			
Activity: _____ Time Sets/reps			

(continued)

Table C-2 *(continued)*

	Month 1	Month 2	Month 3
Week 4			
CARDIO STAMINA			
Activity: _____ Duration Intensity			
Activity: _____ Duration Intensity			
Activity: _____ Duration Intensity			
MUSCLE STRENGTH			
Exercise: _____ Weight Sets/reps			
Exercise: _____ Weight Sets/reps			
Exercise: _____ Weight Sets/reps			
Exercise: _____ Weight Sets/reps			
Exercise: _____ Weight Sets/reps			
Exercise: _____ Weight Sets/reps			

	Month 1	*Month 2*	*Month 3*
Exercise: _____ Weight Sets/reps			
Exercise: _____ Weight Sets/reps			
Exercise: _____ Weight Sets/reps			
Exercise: _____ Weight Sets/reps			
Exercise: _____ Weight Sets/reps			
FLEXIBILITY			
POWER			
Exercise: _____ Time Sets/reps			
Exercise: _____ Time Sets/reps			
Exercise: _____ Time Sets/reps			
Exercise: _____ Time Sets/reps			
Exercise: _____ Time Sets/reps			

(continued)

Table C-2 *(continued)*

	Month 1	Month 2	Month 3
SKILLS Checklist ✓ Easy ✓ Medium ✓ Difficult			
Activity: _____ Time Sets/reps			
Activity: _____ Time Sets/reps			
Activity: _____ Time Sets/reps			
Activity: _____ Time Sets/reps			
Activity: _____ Time Sets/reps			

Yearly Plan

This 12-month schedule allows you to take a long-term perspective on your training by combining as many as four 12-week plans. In order to periodize your training, choose a different *fitness emphasis* to focus on during each 12-week cycle and modify the fitness prescription accordingly. So you might focus on developing cardio stamina in the first cycle and devote more time to the cardio portion of your workouts. In the next cycle, you might concentrate on developing muscle strength. So you might focus on including a wider variety of muscle strength moves, and minimize the amount of cardio you do. In the third cycle you might focus on your sport skills. So you would spend more time doing the agility drills and less on muscle strength moves, and so on. Keep this chart general, and plug in your specific workout details in Table C-1 or Table C-2.

Table C-3	Yearly Log for Year Beginning _____

First Cycle: Months 1-3

Fitness Emphasis:

Cardio stamina

Muscle strength

Flexibility

Power

Skills

Second Cycle: Months 4-6

Fitness Emphasis:

Cardio stamina

Muscle strength

Second Cycle: Months 4-6 (continued)

Fitness Emphasis:

Flexibility

Power

Skills

Third Cycle: Months 7-9

Fitness Emphasis:

Cardio stamina

Muscle strength

Flexibility

Power

Skills

Fourth Cycle: Months 10-12

Fitness Emphasis:

Cardio stamina

Muscle strength

Flexibility

Power

Skills

Index

• C •

• *D* •

• F •

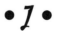

• *W* •

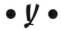

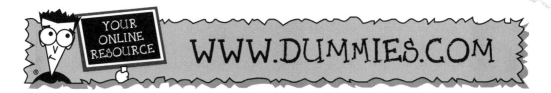

Discover Dummies Online!

The Dummies Web Site is your fun and friendly online resource for the latest information about *For Dummies*® books and your favorite topics. The Web site is the place to communicate with us, exchange ideas with other *For Dummies* readers, chat with authors, and have fun!

Ten Fun and Useful Things You Can Do at www.dummies.com

1. Win free *For Dummies* books and more!
2. Register your book and be entered in a prize drawing.
3. Meet your favorite authors through the IDG Books Worldwide Author Chat Series.
4. Exchange helpful information with other *For Dummies* readers.
5. Discover other great *For Dummies* books you must have!
6. Purchase Dummieswear® exclusively from our Web site.
7. Buy *For Dummies* books online.
8. Talk to us. Make comments, ask questions, get answers!
9. Download free software.
10. Find additional useful resources from authors.

Link directly to these ten fun and useful things at
http://www.dummies.com/10useful

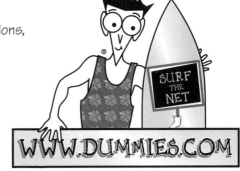

For other technology titles from IDG Books Worldwide, go to
www.idgbooks.com

Not on the Web yet? It's easy to get started with *Dummies 101*®: *The Internet For Windows*® *98* or *The Internet For Dummies*® at local retailers everywhere.

Find other *For Dummies* books on these topics:

Business • Career • Databases • Food & Beverage • Games • Gardening • Graphics • Hardware
Health & Fitness • Internet and the World Wide Web • Networking • Office Suites
Operating Systems • Personal Finance • Pets • Programming • Recreation • Sports
Spreadsheets • Teacher Resources • Test Prep • Word Processing

The IDG Books Worldwide logo is a registered trademark under exclusive license to IDG Books Worldwide, Inc., from International Data Group, Inc. Dummies.com and the ...For Dummies logo are trademarks, and Dummies Man, For Dummies, Dummieswear, and Dummies 101 are registered trademarks of IDG Books Worldwide, Inc. All other trademarks are the property of their respective owners.

IDG BOOKS WORLDWIDE BOOK REGISTRATION

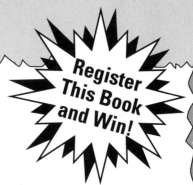

We want to hear from you!

Visit **http://my2cents.dummies.com** to register this book and tell us how you liked it!

- ✔ Get entered in our monthly prize giveaway.

- ✔ Give us feedback about this book — tell us what you like best, what you like least, or maybe what you'd like to ask the author and us to change!

- ✔ Let us know any other *For Dummies®* topics that interest you.

Your feedback helps us determine what books to publish, tells us what coverage to add as we revise our books, and lets us know whether we're meeting your needs as a *For Dummies* reader. You're our most valuable resource, and what you have to say is important to us!

Not on the Web yet? It's easy to get started with *Dummies 101®: The Internet For Windows® 98* or *The Internet For Dummies®* at local retailers everywhere.

Or let us know what you think by sending us a letter at the following address:

For Dummies Book Registration
Dummies Press
10475 Crosspoint Blvd.
Indianapolis, IN 46256

BESTSELLING
BOOK SERIES